MINDFULNESS AND
THE TRANSFORMATION OF DESPAIR

Also Available

For Professionals

Mindfulness-Based Cognitive Therapy for Depression,
Second Edition
*Zindel Segal, Mark Williams,
and John Teasdale*

For General Readers

The Mindful Way through Depression:
Freeing Yourself from Chronic Unhappiness
*Mark Williams, John Teasdale, Zindel Segal,
and Jon Kabat-Zinn*

The Mindful Way Workbook:
An 8-Week Program to Free Yourself
from Depression and Emotional Distress
*John Teasdale, Mark Williams,
and Zindel Segal*

Mindfulness and the Transformation of Despair

Working with People at Risk of Suicide

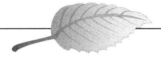

Mark Williams
Melanie Fennell
Thorsten Barnhofer
Rebecca Crane
Sarah Silverton

with Accompanying Audio by
Zindel Segal, Mark Williams, and John Teasdale

THE GUILFORD PRESS
New York   London

© 2015 The Guilford Press
A Division of Guilford Publications, Inc.
370 Seventh Avenue, Suite 1200, New York, NY 10001
www.guilford.com

See p. 334 for terms of use for audio files.

Printed in the United States of America

This book is printed on acid-free paper.

Last digit is print number: 9 8 7 6 5 4 3 2 1

The authors have checked with sources believed to be reliable in their
efforts to provide information that is complete and generally in accord
with the standards of practice that are accepted at the time of publication.
However, in view of the possibility of human error or changes in
behavioral, mental health, or medical sciences, neither the authors, nor
the editor and publisher, nor any other party who has been involved in
the preparation or publication of this work warrants that the information
contained herein is in every respect accurate or complete, and they are not
responsible for any errors or omissions or the results obtained from the use
of such information. Readers are encouraged to confirm the information
contained in this book with other sources.

Library of Congress Cataloging-in-Publication Data
Williams, J. Mark G.
  Mindfulness and the transformation of despair : working with people at
risk of suicide / J. Mark G. Williams [and four others].
     pages   cm
  Includes bibliographical references and index.
  ISBN 978-1-4625-2182-1 (hardback : acid-free paper)
  1. Suicidal behavior—Treatment.   2. Mindfulness-based cognitive
therapy.   3. Psychotherapist and patient.
  RC569.W55 2015
  616.85′84450651—dc23
                                                       2015015978

About the Authors

Mark Williams, DPhil, is Emeritus Professor of Clinical Psychology at the University of Oxford, where he was Wellcome Principal Research Fellow from 2003 to 2012. He collaborated with John Teasdale and Zindel Segal in developing mindfulness-based cognitive therapy (MBCT) to prevent relapse and recurrence in major depression; together, they coauthored *Mindfulness-Based Cognitive Therapy for Depression* (now in its second edition), *The Mindful Way Workbook,* and (with Jon Kabat-Zinn) *The Mindful Way through Depression.* Dr. Williams is a Fellow of the Academy of Medical Sciences and the British Academy. Now retired, he continues to train mindfulness teachers around the world.

Melanie Fennell, PhD, is a Founding Fellow of the Oxford Cognitive Therapy Centre, where she is now an Associate Trainer. She is also an Associate Trainer at the Oxford Mindfulness Centre. As a research clinician in the University of Oxford Department of Psychiatry, she contributed to the development of evidence-based treatments for depression and anxiety disorders, including MBCT. She developed and led the Oxford Diploma in Cognitive Therapy, the Oxford Diploma/MSc in Advanced Cognitive Therapy Studies, and (with Mark Williams) the Oxford Master of Studies Program in Mindfulness-Based Cognitive Therapy. Dr. Fennell is an Honorary Fellow of the British Association of Behavioural and Cognitive Psychotherapies (BABCP) and was voted "Most Influential Female UK Cognitive Therapist" by the BABCP's membership in 2002.

Thorsten Barnhofer, PhD, is a Heisenberg Fellow at Charité, the joint medical faculty of the Free University of Berlin and Humboldt University, where he investigates the neural mechanisms of mindfulness training in the treatment and prevention of depression. Previously, he worked in Professor Williams's group at the Oxford Department of Psychiatry, where he was involved in research on MBCT for suicidal and chronic depression. A cognitive-behavioral therapist and yoga teacher, Dr. Barnhofer regularly teaches MBCT training workshops and retreats for mental health professionals.

Rebecca Crane, PhD, MA, DipCot, is Director of the Centre for Mindfulness Research and Practice at Bangor University in Wales. She previously worked in the mental health field as an occupational therapist and an integrative counselor. Dr. Crane teaches and trains internationally in both MBCT and mindfulness-based stress reduction (MBSR), and is a certified MBSR teacher with the Center for Mindfulness in Medicine, Health Care, and Society at the University of Massachusetts Medical School.

Sarah Silverton, DipCot, MEd, teaches at the Centre for Mindfulness Research and Practice at Bangor University, Wales. She has extensive experience as an occupational therapist, counselor, and mindfulness teacher and trainer. She is the author of *The Mindfulness Breakthrough*.

Zindel Segal, PhD, is Distinguished Professor of Psychology in Mood Disorders at the University of Toronto–Scarborough. His research focuses on vulnerability to and prevention of mood disorders, and he has published more than 10 books and 150 scientific publications. Dr. Segal is a founding Fellow of the Academy of Cognitive Therapy and advocates for the relevance of mindfulness-based clinical care in psychiatry and mental health.

John Teasdale, PhD, held a Special Scientific Appointment with the United Kingdom Medical Research Council's Cognition and Brain Sciences Unit in Cambridge. Dr. Teasdale is a founding Fellow of the Academy of Cognitive Therapy and a Fellow of the British Academy and the Academy of Medical Sciences. He also is a recipient of the Distinguished Scientist Award from Division 12 (Society of Clinical Psychology) of the American Psychological Association. Since retiring, Dr. Teasdale has taught insight meditation internationally.

Acknowledgments

There are numerous people who contributed to the making of this book.

We are deeply grateful for the long collaboration and friendship with John Teasdale and Zindel Segal, whose work on the psychological theory underlying mindfulness practice has provided a much-needed bridge between ancient wisdom and modern science, an understanding that led to mindfulness-based cognitive therapy (MBCT), which remains the foundation for the work we report in this book.

We are continually grateful for the seminal work undertaken by Jon Kabat-Zinn in originating mindfulness-based stress reduction (MBSR), and for the teaching team at the Center for Mindfulness in Medicine, Health Care, and Society at the University of Massachusetts Medical School, who have graciously and generously supported the development of MBCT—particular appreciation goes to Ferris Urbanowski, Pamela Erdmann, Melissa Blacker, Saki Santorelli, Elana Rosenbaum, and Florence Meleo-Meyer.

Our colleagues Catherine Crane and Keith Hawton have been particularly crucial anchors throughout the research reported in the book. We thank others in the research team—Kate Brennan, Caroline Creasey, Danielle Duggan, Catrin Eames, Mariel Jones, Kate Muse, Ann Hackmann, Adele Krusche, Sholto Radford, Isabelle Rudolf Von Rohr, Ian and Daphne Russell, Dhruvi Shah, Wendy Swift, Yongzhong Sun, Shirley Thomas, Elaine Weatherley-Jones, and Christopher Whitaker.

Colleagues within the Centre for Mindfulness Research and Practice in Bangor, Wales, gave important support to us during the trial. Jody Mardula took over the leadership of the center at this time to enable the research. Judith Soulsby, Eluned Gold, Sharon Hadley, and David Shannon were also generous in their support of this work.

The research was supported by Grant No. GR067797 from the Wellcome Trust to Mark Williams and Ian Russell, and we are particularly grateful to Candace Hassall, Louise Williams, and John Williams of Wellcome for their generous guidance and support over many years. Our personal and technical support came from the University of Oxford and Bangor University.

We are grateful for the warm hospitality we received in the beautiful setting of Hawkstone Hall in Shropshire, where most of the book was written.

We thank our families, who gave us the space to write.

Most importantly, we thank our participants for taking the courageous step to join an MBCT group. We are grateful to them for allowing us to reflect their experiences in this book. Many expressed a wish to join the research to support personal learning, but also to contribute to collective learning so that in the future people who are experiencing despair can receive the best support possible. We are glad of their generosity, and are also delighted that for many the work has been transformational.

Contents

CHAPTER 1

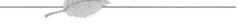

Introduction

It is one of the most difficult and painful conversations that takes place between a person seeking help for his or her psychological difficulties and the therapist, counselor, or teacher to whom he or she has come to see. For when questions about their life history have been asked, about their family and work, about what brings them here, about signs and symptoms of the depression, hopelessness, and mental pain that can accompany any physical or psychological problem, there needs to be a question about suicide: "Have things ever got to the point that you've considered ending it all; that life just wasn't worth living anymore; that even suicide would be better than carrying on like this?" He or she may have told no one, and yet feel a huge burden of guilt about harboring such thoughts.

There are many different ways of asking, but eventually the issue has to be addressed, especially if the person is or has been clinically depressed. Half of those who become depressed will have recurrent thoughts of death or suicide, but while any psychological problem increases the risk of suicide—anxiety or panic, bipolar disorder, posttraumatic stress disorder (PTSD), schizophrenia—it is the sense of depression and helplessness that comes with these problems that exacerbates the risk that someone may take his or her own life. Depression and hopelessness form the "final common pathway" for suicidal feelings and behavior, and it is suicidal depression and hopelessness that this book is about.

The approach to those at risk of suicide described in this book arose from a larger quest to help those suffering from depression in general. Depression is consistently ranked in the top four disorders in terms of global disease burden and has been described as a significant global challenge for the 21st century (Collins et al., 2011). Twenty percent of the population will be seriously depressed at some point in their lives—over a billion people across the globe—and it blights the lives of people whether they live in high-, middle-, or low-income countries (World Health Organization, 2008). Wherever it strikes, depression erodes the well-being and quality of life of sufferers and their families and profoundly impairs people's ability to function in their day-to-day personal, social, and working lives. But it is a hidden scar—few people talk about it as openly as they would about other causes of disability.

In 1993, Zindel Segal, John Teasdale and Mark Williams set out to find a way of understanding the factors that increase risk of depression and then how that risk might be reduced. Originally they had intended to base their preventative approach on cognitive therapy, but their own personal experience and new scientific findings about what processes underlie the maintenance of high risk in depression convinced them that there was more to be discovered than was contained in their existing cognitive theories and therapies. Learning from Marsha Linehan's use of mindfulness (a key feature of her dialectical behavior therapy for people with a diagnosis of borderline personality disorder), and Jon Kabat-Zinn's pioneering work at UMass Medical Center on mindfulness-based stress reduction (MBSR), they proposed a psychological model to explain why mindfulness training, with its emphasis on changing *modes* of mind, might be helpful for people who repeatedly get stuck in recurrent and toxic patterns of mind.

But what is "mindfulness"? The word "mindfulness" is a translation of an ancient Pali word, originally meaning memory or nonforgetfulness. In the Buddhist writings it came to mean "lucid awareness" (Bodhi, 2011). In its more common usage in recent clinical literature, it has come to mean the awareness that emerges as a by-product of cultivating three related skills: (1) intentionally paying attention to moment-by-moment events as they unfold in the internal and external world; (2) noticing habitual reactions to such events, often characterized by aversion or attachment (commonly resulting in rumination and avoidance); and (3) cultivating the ability to respond to events, and to reactions to them, with an attitude of open curiosity and compassion. Mindfulness is traditionally cultivated by meditation in which people learn to pay attention in each moment with full intentionality and with friendly interest. When people practice such meditation for any length of time, a number of qualities of their experience change. People say they feel more aware or awake, feel calmer and are more able to see clearly and gain freedom from their own emotional patterns and habits, free to be more compassionate to themselves and to others. The early research trials conducted by Kabat-Zinn and his colleagues had shown that this approach could be highly effective for patients who suffered long-term physical health conditions that had been destroying the quality of their lives (Kabat-Zinn, 2013).

Segal, Williams, and Teasdale recognized that mindfulness training might be the key to preventing depression. The research trial they carried out at the University of Cambridge (England), the University of Toronto (Canada), and Bangor University (Wales) showed that for those who had suffered three or more previous episodes of depression, mindfulness-based cognitive therapy (MBCT) reduced the rates of relapse by between 40 and 50% (Teasdale et al., 2000).

At that time, they were cautiously optimistic that mindfulness could pay a role in the reduction of risk of depression, but believed that such an approach might be of interest to a minority of clinicians. In 2002, they published a book that told the story of their research, their false starts and reversals, and what they eventually discovered. To their surprise, the book, *Mindfulness-Based Cognitive Therapy for Depression: A New Approach to Preventing Relapse* (Segal et al., 2002), was widely read and became highly influential. It transformed the whole landscape of clinical practice, changing both the way people understood depression and how best to prevent it, and then went on to have a wide impact on the field of evidence-based approaches to other serious psychological conditions.

Mindfulness and Suicidality

But there were gnawing questions being asked again and again: Can mindfulness be used for the most vulnerable people, that is, for those who have a history of severe adversity? What if people get *more* upset because mindfulness has made them more aware of their difficulties? What if they have a risk for suicide? Wouldn't it be unethical to encourage people to do a practice that might end up with them becoming *more* aware of suicidal thoughts and feelings? Williams had long been concerned about those people who become so depressed that they consider suicide as their only option. His colleagues and coworkers in the International Association for Suicide Prevention had shown that across the globe each year, around one million people commit suicide. Suicide claims more lives than war. There was an urgent need to help, but few clues about how best to do so.

In January 2003 Williams moved from Bangor University to the University of Oxford to begin a 10-year research program as a Wellcome Trust Principal Research Fellow, setting up a team that would be able to investigate whether the psychological processes underlying mindfulness, that enable it to help prevent recurrence in depression, could also apply to those who suffered depression so severely that they became suicidal. Oxford was the center of choice since this is where Keith Hawton had been working for many years at the forefront of research into suicide and suicidal behavior. Here was an opportunity to deepen our understanding of the particular vulnerabilities of people who had suffered so much throughout their lives that they were persistently thinking of ending it all. Could mindfulness help them? Ultimately, the team would have to carry out a research trial to see whether and for whom mindfulness might be helpful. But before that, there was a lot of work to be done to clarify exactly what made some people suicidal. Only if they could understand the factors that trigger and maintain suicidal thinking and behavior could they begin to see what might help.

This book is the story of what they discovered, and about the impact these new understandings had on their approach to MBCT. It would affect their view of how to train new therapists in MBCT, and how to assess competence in teaching it. But most importantly, the research would show them how best to offer MBCT to those suffering not only from suicidal depression but also from other difficulties that have chronic histories and persistent symptoms.

Overview of This Book

We have divided the chapters in this book into four parts. In Part I, we cover the research and theoretical background. Chapter 2 describes the "cry of pain" model of suicidality, and how hopelessness and despair can be switched on very suddenly under certain circumstances—when a person feels defeated and believes deeply that he or she has no escape route. Chapter 3 goes into more detail about what we found when we tested these theories in the laboratory. We see the science behind suicide risk—examining the difficulty that some people have in bringing to mind positive images of the future and then the way people differ, one from another, in how reactive they are to small changes in mood. Reactivity not only encompasses negative themes but also rumination and avoidance. More specifically, in those at risk of suicide, reactivity includes graphic images of suicide that, while being intrusive and disturbing for some sufferers, are comforting for a few. Finally we see how subtle changes in the way people recall their personal past (autobiographical memory) affects their reactivity to the present.

If we hope that the mindfulness approach will be taken seriously by those who are most vulnerable, we have to explain to them why mindfulness training might be appropriate for them to try. Chapter 4 offers a framework a clinician can use for answering the patient's question "Will it work for me . . . and how can it help?"

Part II moves from the laboratory and into the clinic, describing the practical application of the Part I research. Chapter 5 examines how we can best assess suicidal vulnerability in order to ensure that we know as much as we can about the risks, and do not do harm. In Chapter 6, we tell the story of how a pilot clinical trial to test our ideas revealed important factors about who drops out before the end of a MBCT course, and describe how we elaborated the preclass interview so as to enhance engagement in the program. We take the learning from this into Chapters 7–14, in which we describe, session by session, the specific changes we made to the original MBCT for depression protocol, and how our participants experienced these changes. These chapters go into detail about the way MBCT can be offered to those in whom strong suicidal thoughts and actions can be easily activated. If it is true that transformation can come only by our "turning toward difficulties," how can this be done in a way that provides a place of genuine safety for participants in the class?

Chapter 15 summarizes the MBCT program by "listening" to the dialogues that take place in the class between teacher and a single participant. It is out of this dialogue following each meditation (often called "inquiry") that much or most learning takes place.

Part III moves into considering the crucial role of the teacher. In Chapter 16, we turn to the controversial question of how we assess the quality of teaching in mindfulness-based interventions. For any evidence-based therapy, it is important to know that what is taught week by week is faithful to the intentions of the approach—that the teaching covers the curriculum, and is taught at a certain level of competence. These issues are not confined to research trial contexts. If we want to disseminate mindfulness teaching to trainees, we need to have a clear understanding of the skills and processes we are conveying as a framework for training and supervision. So the question arises: How can we consistently and reliably assess competence and adherence (the "integrity" of the teaching)? The answer to this question is not simple, because the process of teaching and learning within any mindfulness-based intervention is subtle, and in a large part arises implicitly through the process rather than by covering an explicit curriculum. So assessment of teaching has also to address the "hidden curriculum," that is, how teachers embody the learning in their own way of being. This chapter considers the issues of mindfulness-based teaching integrity, what it is, how it develops over time, and how it can be assessed. Chapter 17 approaches teaching from a different and complementary angle, focusing on the experience of the teacher "from the inside." How can teachers best remain true to the curriculum and intentions of the approach when working with the most vulnerable patients? In particular, the chapter explores the challenges of teaching a manualized, protocol-based program, and the need to balance adherence to the particular, defined curriculum of MBCT, on the one hand, with flexibility and responsiveness to participants, on the other.

Finally, we move to Part IV. In Chapter 18, we summarize the previous chapters, and reveal what we found when we tested MBCT in a large randomized controlled trial—and what the results show us about how to treat the most vulnerable patients, including the best approach to dealing skillfully with reactions of extreme suicidal despair. We place our findings in the context of trials of MBCT that have been published more recently and that inform our view of how to move forward with this evidence-based approach. In sum, by the end of the book, we shall have identified the practical implications for mindfulness teachers, in terms of how they can assess would-be participants' suitability for MBCT, and how to shape its planning and delivery, remaining faithful to the protocol without undue rigidity or fear, as well as drawing out the implications for teachers for sustaining their own practice and continuing their own training.

How to Use This Book

No single book on mindfulness stands alone. Each one work contributes its own piece to a long-standing and worldwide body of knowledge, understanding, and practice. This book is no exception: it is intended to complement the standard MBCT manual of Segal, Williams, and Teasdale (2013) both in terms of describing its adaptation for highly vulnerable patients, and also in providing additional information on recent general developments that are relevant from a broader perspective, such as the definition and assessment of teacher competency. The book is not a "manual," and we would caution against any teacher or therapist imagining that mindfulness alone will "cure" suicidal thoughts and behavior. Segal and colleagues are very clear about knowing the limits of our competence when any of us are working with trauma and serious mental distress, and we endorse their advice about the training required to work in this field (Segal et al., 2013, pp. 420–421).

The book follows an inherent logic, and it would be best to read it in the sequence presented. In this way, the modifications to the MBCT program and its delivery become understandable from a background of research findings, and the advice on how to implement the program week by week is informed by our best current knowledge. We often recommend that teachers reread the relevant chapter in the book before teaching a particular session, not only in order to remind themselves of the structure of the session, but also to reacquaint themselves with its broader theme and the characteristic responses that may recur. Being prepared in terms of the "hidden curriculum" may be particularly important when working with highly vulnerable patients, so we have laid out key issues in Part II (Chapters 7–14), session by session. To support the implementation of the MBCT program, we have made available audio recordings of practice exercises from the second edition of *Mindfulness-Based Cognitive Therapy for Depression* (Segal et al., 2013), which can be streamed directly from the Web or downloaded in MP3 format. Participants find the recordings helpful, especially when they are getting started in practicing mindfulness. Teachers can access these tracks at *www.guilford.com/williams6-materials*. Finally, in the later chapters focusing on the experience of the teacher, we intend to convey a sense of what is important psychologically in helping teachers to respond with understanding, compassion, and care to suicidality and despair in MBCT and in other settings.

We hope the book will serve as a helpful resource not only for those teaching MBCT to highly vulnerable patients but also for those who might not be involved in teaching mindfulness in a mental health setting but nonetheless find that they, or those who come to them for help, struggle with suicidality, and despair.

Suicide is a tragedy that affects many of us, families, friends and colleagues of those who have taken their lives, leaving behind feelings of shame, anger, loneliness, and sorrow. As therapists, clinicians, counselors, or mindfulness teachers, we need to deepen and extend our understanding of the field in general and our vulnerable clients or participants in particular. We dedicate this book to all those whose lives have been touched by such a tragedy. May it bring fresh perspectives, courage, and wisdom for those working with people at risk of suicide.

PART I

THEORETICAL AND RESEARCH BACKGROUND

CHAPTER 2

The Origins of Despair

An Evolutionary Perspective

Cathy did not really understand how she ended up in the hospital. Well, of course, she knew that she'd had a huge argument with a close friend, that she'd gone home by herself and started to drink, and not gone to another friend's wedding on the weekend, making some excuse about the illness that was going round the office. But that had been 4 days ago . . . she'd been at work since and got on with her life. Then old feelings of loneliness and the sheer pointlessness of life had begun to overwhelm her in the evenings. Here she was, in her 30s, with no real friends, living alone, a job she didn't really enjoy, and a past that was blighted by a recurring sense of failure. She had always wondered how other people really "did" life . . . how did they "make themselves happy" when, to her, there never seemed to be anything to be happy about. She never seemed to be on the same wavelength as other people. Worse than this, she seemed to make everyone else around her unhappy.

That Thursday, when it happened, she had come home from work as usual, with a crushing headache, and gone to the cupboard to get some painkillers. She opened the cupboard and saw the pills, and also the antidepressants she'd been prescribed last year but never taken, and the very strong painkillers her mother had left by mistake last year when she'd stayed. Suddenly it occurred to her, like a light going on somewhere in her head—she didn't have to put up with this. If she removed herself from the world, everyone else would be better off. She'd stop being a burden to others, and stop the pain she was finding unbearable.

Everything that happened after that was a blur. Here she was, in the hospital with a drip in her arm, with her parents sitting by her bedside looking completely defeated, some flowers from her recently married friend on the table beside her, and a constant voice in her head telling her how stupid she'd been—she couldn't even succeed at taking her own life. The ER physician said she had been close to death, very close indeed. It was a miracle she was alive, he'd said. Cathy did not agree. She'd wanted to die, and now did not know what she wanted.

The Challenge for Therapists

Cathy's story is repeated thousands of times a day across the world. How can we understand how to prevent episodes like these? Suicide and suicidal behavior are complex phenomena—understandable at the level of sociology, psychology, and biology. Understanding who is most at risk and whether people can be helped to live a life that is worth living, so that such overwhelming feelings can be handled in a way that is not so destructive, is a huge challenge.

Let us first make clear how we see the issue from an ethical point of view. It could be argued that suicide is a free act, that no one else should interfere with a person's right to end his or her own life. Here are some views that we have heard expressed by clinicians, any or all of which would undermine our motivation to help:

- The causes of suicide have nothing to do with mental illness: it is an illness of society.
- Suicide is a matter that should be left for the individual to decide.
- Suicide is too rare for us to predict.
- Suicidal individuals rarely contact professional services. Even if they do contact us, they do not talk about their suicidal intent.
- Patients who talk about suicide rarely go on to do it.
- Focusing on suicide in the clinical interview only increases risk.

Contrast these attitudes with some alternatives:

- Those at risk of suicide come to us in our professional capacity to get help.
- Even though they have thought about or even planned suicide

for many weeks, months or years, they are still alive—something is keeping them from dying.

- Most people, even when very hopeless, are usually ambivalent about suicide, and we have a responsibility to encourage the wish to live.
- Suicidal clients have already talked with relatives and friends, and we may well be their last port of call.
- Most people who attempt suicide, and who die by suicide, are depressed at the time they do it. Depression involves a style of thinking that makes suicide seem the only option.
- Things can improve in a most unexpected way even in the case of people facing enormous adverse odds.
- It is for us to assume that change for the better is always possible.

We agree with this latter stance. By whatever route a person has come to us, here he or she is—still alive despite everything. We are committed to offering this person, right now, a way in which he or she can come to see for him- or herself that life may surprise him or her with its possibilities even when all seems to point to despair.

Systematic reviews of the research (National Institute for Health and Clinical Excellence, 2011) show that, although there remains uncertainty about which treatments are most effective, those that include clarification of the patterns that underlie interpersonal difficulties in order to improve the availability of problem-solving options carry some promise. Yet there is general agreement that there is much we do not know. For treatments to progress further, we need to understand clearly and precisely the psychological processes that underlie both long-term vulnerability, what factors from time to time activate these processes, and how activation can be followed by a swift downturn in mood, exacerbated by reawakened negative thinking patterns, and culminating for some in a spiral into suicidal despair. Our approach is based on the observation that most suicidal thinking and behavior occur in the context of hopelessness and despair about the future. Suicidal feelings can come about very rapidly, but most often they occur in the context of an episode of depression, even if the depression has been successfully hidden from the view of family or friends.

In the book *Cry of Pain,* Williams (1997, 2014) describes the way in which we might best understand suicidal feeling and behavior. The title was chosen deliberately as an attempt to answer those who tend to dismiss suicidal behavior (often now called deliberate self-harm) as a "cry for help." The expression "cry for help" had been coined by, amongst others, Erwin Stengel (1964) in his book *Suicide and Attempted Suicide*. He had talked about the "appeal function" of such behavior, but this description was widely misunderstood, as if he meant that suicidal behavior is *only* a cry for help. Even now, many suicidal acts are dismissed as "mere" cries for help, as if a communication motive was incompatible with a serious attempt to end life, and as if the self-damaging act did not represent a deeper anguish that needs to be taken very seriously indeed. In fact, Stengel was drawing attention to the fact that a suicidal act shares with physical illness the characteristic of drawing out from others a wish to come to the aid of the person in need.

The "cry of pain" perspective was intended instead to capture the way in which any behavior can have a communication outcome without communication being the main motive. An animal caught in a trap cries with pain. The cry is brought about by the pain, but may also communicate distress in a way that will affect the behavior of other animals. Suicidal behavior may be overtly communicative in a minority of cases, but mainly it is "elicited" by the pain of a situation with which the person cannot cope—a cry of pain first, and only then a cry for help.

The "cry for help" idea had another unintended consequence. Because it was limited to nonfatal suicide attempts, it contributed to a widening of the gap between how people thought about nonfatal suicide attempts and suicide. As pointed out in *Cry of Pain* (Williams, 1997, 2014), attempted suicide and completed suicide are very closely related. Both affect the more socially disadvantaged, and the motives for both completed and attempted suicide share many features. For example, anger and communication issues can be found both in suicide and in acts of self-harm that do not have a fatal outcome, and even relatively low-risk "suicidal ideas" (which often do not lead to suicidal behavior) may be dominated by the theme of escape and death rather than communicating feelings with another person.

You can see this mixture of feelings in Cathy's experience—and she might have easily ended up as one of the 38,000 people a year who kill themselves in the United States (*www.cdc.gov/nchs/fastats/suicide.*

htm)—contributing to 800,000 suicide deaths worldwide each year (*www.who.int/mental_health/prevention/suicide*). The number of people who harm themselves intentionally but who do not die is staggering. A recent population-based study showed that almost 19% of 16- to 17-year-olds had engaged in some self-harm on at least one occasion (Kidger, Heron, Lewis, Evans, & Gunnell, 2012). Most of this behavior is without clear suicide intent, but if there is history of suicidal behavior in close friends or family, then the behavior is more likely to have a wish to die in its mix of motives (Hargus, Hawton, & Rodham, 2009).

Although this behavior seems to describe extreme reactions to stress, we suggest that such moments arise in all our lives, whether externally or internally generated. We all live on a spectrum in which helplessness and loss, illness and death, are never far away. Human minds have myriad ways in which we can find ourselves trapped, feeling momentarily paralyzed. For some, such moments of despair can lead to a sense of wanting to exit the world, to escape from the self.

Those who feel despairing and suicidal often live (or have lived) in very difficult circumstances, or have come to understand their world in ways that make them feel helpless and confused. Some may encounter these mind-states because they have a genetic disposition toward large and unpredictable mood swings. But whatever factors contribute to these periods of deep despair, the cry of pain view suggests that all of them will ultimately have their effects on people through a final common pathway: the feeling of being totally defeated combined with the feeling that there is no escape.

Can Existing Psychological Treatment Help?

Despite a great deal of research on suicidal ideas, planning, and behavior, identifying ways to help such patients in order to reduce risk of repetition has proven difficult. As we have mentioned, the recent systematic review of the research studies to date showed that there remains considerable uncertainty about which approaches are most effective (National Institute for Health and Care Excellence [NICE], 2011). This uncertainty arises from the fact that even the best cognitive or problem-based approaches either report only modest success or have not been replicated. Even in the case of cognitive therapy (CT), there is a paucity of studies showing effectiveness. Brown et al. studied participants who were highly socially vulnerable; over 40% had an income of $8,000 or less, and 66% were unemployed or disabled (Brown et al., 2005). They found that many people failed to turn up for appointments or turned up at the wrong time and could not be seen in the usual clinic, where the therapists were engaged in other clinical duties. So they radically changed what they were doing, introducing case managers for every patient in the study, who became responsible for keeping in touch with clients, giving out bus tokens, conducting home visits, picking up some patients in cars, arranging community voicemail facilities, using the Philadelphia Homeless Database to track patients, and identifying at the outset some contact people who would be likely to know where the patient was at any time. The study found a drop from 38% to 20% in repeated suicidal behavior in the period following the CT intervention. However, there are no more studies of this type, so we cannot know if it could be replicated by others. Attempts to use day-patient treatment (Bateman & Fonagy, 2008) and CT (Davidson, Tyrer, Norrie, Palmer, & Tyrer, 2010) for reducing suicidal behavior in patients with a diagnosis of personality disorder have proven moderately successful, but need replicating.

Linehan's (1993) dialectical behavior therapy (DBT) for those with borderline personality disorder is an exception. DBT combines weekly individual and weekly group therapy over a 1-year period. It uses treatment strategies from behavioral, cognitive, and supportive psychotherapies. A behavioral/problem-solving component focuses on enhancing capability, generating alternative ways of coping, and clarifying and managing contingencies—all with the emphasis on the "here-and-now." The "dialectical" of its title lies in its emphasis on balancing *acceptance* of (seeing clearly) the stresses that exist in the environment, on the one hand, with the need to *change* how to approach them, on the other. The theme is encouraging clients to really grasp how things are ("grasp" or "take in" is the root meaning of the word *accept*). Once a person has understood things clearly and deeply as they really are, they are more able to step back from them temporarily to see what things may be changed.

The individual therapy prioritizes themes related to suicidal behavior. Linehan believes this is a critical part of the therapy. She asserts that newly trained therapists too easily avoid explicit discussion of suicidal thoughts, urges, and behavior. The client needs to learn that help for other problems can only be discussed when the self-harm behavior has been faced directly and then brought under control.

Weekly group skills training, which lasts for 2½ hours a session, focuses on themes of *interpersonal problem solving, distress tolerance, mindfulness*, and *emotional regulation.*

Studies to assess the effectiveness of DBT have been encouraging.[*] Altogether, they constitute impressive evidence that this approach provides a major source of hope for many people with some of the most intractable social and emotional problems.

But apart from the extensive research by Linehan on those with serious personality disorder, there are no treatment approaches that have been found to be effective in reducing suicidal behavior and then been replicated in further studies. Knowing how best to understand and help with suicidal feelings that arise in the context of serious recurrent depression has not been addressed systematically. There is simply not sufficient research on how best to understand and treat suicidal ideation, planning, and behavior to be sure that we have done our best for those who come to us for help. Treatments have evolved as pragmatic approaches, but until recent research on the cognitive mechanisms underlying problem-solving deficits, these treatments proceeded in the absence of any understanding of the psychology of despair and what happens to the capacity to problem-solve in its presence.

The Cry of Pain

In the light of the paucity of theory and evidence to guide our efforts in developing new understandings and treatment approaches, we returned to the research of evolutionary psychologists, who have important insights to give on the circumstances in which all living beings give up and become helpless in the face of stressors. We are deeply indebted to Gilbert's (1989) *Human Nature and Suffering* for the following way of looking at depression and powerlessness in general, and suicidal feelings in particular.

---

[*]Ten studies have evaluated the efficacy of DBT for suicidal patients with BPD—nine of which are discussed in the U.K. NICE (2009) guidelines for BPD.

Consider the behavior of birds establishing their territories. If birds meet within a single territory, they engage in aggressive displays. One wins, the other loses. The loser flies away to find another territory. It suffers little ill effects from its encounter. But if this meeting occurs in a limited territory, in a cage or other circumstance in which the defeated bird cannot escape, it is a different story. Here is a description of what happens then:

> Its behavior becomes entirely changed. Deeply depressed in spirit, humbled, with drooping wings and head in the dust, it is overcome with paralysis, although one cannot detect any physical injury. The bird's resistance now seems broken, and in some cases the effects of the psychological conditions are so strong that the bird sooner or later comes to grief. (Schjelderup-Ebbe, 1985, quoted in Price & Sloman, 1987, p. 87S)

While it is dangerous to jump too readily from nonhuman animals to human behavior, there are good reasons to allow such observations to help in generating *hypotheses* about what psychosocial and biological processes might underlie human behavior. Note certain things from the bird example. First, the defeated bird's behavior occurs in the absence of physical damage. Second, the defeat itself is not sufficient to trigger the response. If a defeated bird can escape to another territory, it shows no ill effect. It is the combination of *defeat* and the *lack of escape* that is needed for the reaction to occur (what Gilbert calls "arrested flight"). Third, an animal that is showing such a learned helplessness reaction can recover if removed from the situation, but it will take some time, and longer if the animal is prone to react with helplessness to stressors. These features of the defeated bird's behavior suggested to many that what the defeat has done is to trigger an evolutionary primitive biological process, a biological process that then takes time to reverse. So there is a third factor in the equation in addition to "defeat" and "no escape." There is the presence (or absence) of *rescue factors* that will determine how long lasting the reaction is. These ideas have also been explored in more detail by Rory O'Connor (2003), who has added the helpful suggestion that the factors that increase risk of suicidal *ideas* (e.g., a sense of not belonging any more, of being a burden, and having no sense of there being a positive future) may be distinct from those that increase the risk of actual suicidal *behavior* (e.g., impulsivity, high intention to act and actual planning, access to the means, and imitation of others [O'Connor, 2011]).

The "cry of pain" hypothesis (Williams, 1997, 2014) uses arrested flight as its central component. It suggests that biological scripts similar to those switched on by real defeat for the bird can be switched on in humans by *psychological* representations of defeat. According to this model, suicidal behavior represents the response to a situation that has these three components: defeat, no escape, and no rescue (real or imagined). So if someone is exposed to (and sensitive to) social signals that represent defeat, no escape, and no rescue, he or she is likely to be vulnerable to the triggering of primitive "helplessness" biological processes. Let us look at each of these psychological processes in turn to see if there exists evidence to support the model.

Sensitivity to Signals of Defeat

In looking for evidence of a psychological process that renders a person particularly sensitive to stimuli signaling possible or actual defeat or "loser status," our research began in the 1980s with work on attentional bias. There is a well-described phenomenon called "perceptual popout" in which a stimulus that is of great interest to a person (a current concern) appears to jump out at him/her. This explains one's ability to hear one's own name, even across a crowded room at a party (hence called the "cocktail party phenomenon"). As such, it is a normal perceptual/ attentional process (Kahneman, 2012, would call it a feature of System 1), ensuring that one does not miss information that is important for one's well-being. It occurs when one is buying a new car (suddenly one sees many such types of car on the road) or buying a house (the salience of "For Sale" signs increases dramatically).

Research has found that the way in which such salient items "pop out" is almost completely involuntary (see Williams, Watts, MacLeod, & Mathews, 1997, Ch. 4 and 5, for review). For someone who is sensitive to failure (or has been made sensitive by his or her circumstances), the world will appear to have many more aspects that refer to defeat and rejection. At exactly the point in their lives when they need relief from stress and pressure, the attentional bias causes them instead to be bombarded with stimuli signaling that they are "losers."

To see if this process occurs in suicidal people, we used the emotional Stroop task. In this task, the person sees a series of words that are printed in colored inks. Their task is to call out the colors in which the words are printed, as fast as possible but making as few errors as possible. A large number of studies had shown that, if the *meaning* of the word is salient (i.e., tends to "pop out") there will be interference with the naming of the color. For example, someone who is afraid of spiders, when shown the word "spider" written in red ink and told to name the color, will not be able to avoid seeing the word. He or she will be relatively slow to name the color of those words that are personally salient. Because such attentional popout is involuntary, it is difficult for a person to avoid slowing down color naming on words that carry special significance. Our results showed clear evidence of attentional bias. Overdose patients were slowed down in their color naming of words signaling defeat and rejection, and, given their recent history, particularly slowed down by words concerning an overdose.

We suggest that such involuntary hypersensitivity to stimuli signaling "loser" status increases the risk that the defeat response will be triggered. This brings us to our second psychological process.

The Sense of Being Trapped

Recall that the defeat (or signals of defeat) was not enough to trigger the full-blown reaction. There also needed to be the sense of "no escape," "entrapment," or "arrested flight." As Kahneman (2012) has pointed out, once System 1 has alerted a person to something he or she needs to attend to, the slower, more effortful System 2 gets to work to analyze it. It is here things can go terribly wrong.

Numerous studies have pointed out the importance of problem-solving difficulties in suicidal patients. Our analysis suggests that problem-solving difficulties in themselves are not important. It is the fact that they indicate to the person "there is no escape" that makes them significant. If one cannot define a problem, or if one cannot generate ideas about how to solve it, then the sense of being trapped is never likely to be far away.

Duggan (2008) examined this issue in some detail. She wanted to know how much repetition of suicidal behavior could be predicted by difficulties in problem solving. She recruited 50 patients from a hospital in Oxford who had been admitted following deliberate self-harm, and who had been in the hospital at least once before after a similar event. She assessed a number of aspects of their psychological profile and history, and found that a measure of their *effectiveness in solving interpersonal problems* predicted whether they came to the hospital again for treatment after deliberately harming themselves over the next 16 months. Her conclusion was consistent with an emerging clinical literature suggesting that impaired problem solving is a critical factor in rendering someone vulnerable.

How Do Such Problem-Solving Difficulties Arise?

Our research suggests that a critical aspect of a person's ability to solve current problems is his or her ability to access past events from his or her life. But not any type of memory will do. Quite by chance, some years ago, we discovered that people give different types of memory responses when asked about their past depending on whether they are depressed, and on whether they have a history of trauma.

Imagine being in one of our experiments: we ask you to remember any event from your past that made you *happy* (or *angry*, or *surprised*, or *safe*—or any number of other positive, negative, or neutral words can be used as well). We say that the event you recall could come from the recent past, or from a long time ago, but it should be a *specific* event, something that happened that took less than a day. It does not have to be unique: "having coffee with a friend last Friday" would do, but saying "having coffee with friends every Friday" would not, because it does not pick out one particular time. In fact, people normally have little difficulty in retrieving an example: *Happy*: "when I got a high grade in history"; "when Anya brought me a bunch of flowers from the garden"; "the day we got our new kitten."

We found that suicidal patients tend to give a type of response which, though similar in some ways, differs in one important respect. Take, for example, the following responses: Happy: "when people give me presents"; "getting good grades at school"; "taking the dog for a walk every Sunday when we used to live near the beach."

Notice that these do not describe a specific event. Instead they are summaries or "categories" of a number of events—hence we call these "categoric memories." It is as if these patients have "stopped short" of retrieving the specific event. Note that we are not asking them to recall events that are difficult or traumatic. It is possible that such patients suffer a bombardment of intrusive memories from the past, and have adopted a strategy of overgeneral memory to regulate their emotions. They stop short of recalling specifics (positive as well as negative) lest doing so brings up an event that might remind them of a difficulty or a trauma. But there may not have been any trauma in the past. Some people tend to avoid emotion, and if they think that a personal memory might bring up emotion, they tend to switch to more overgeneral retrieval (Debeer, Raes, Williams, & Hermans, 2011). The problem for others is exacerbated when their attempts to recall events from the past simply activate ruminative thinking, such as "I can't be happy." Under these circumstances, the rumination may be so all-absorbing that they may not even have the cognitive capacity to remember the instructions of the task; they are now "caught" in their own processes, and cannot focus on recalling what they had been asked to recall (Dalgleish et al., 2007)

Several studies, on both suicidal patients and patients suffering from depression, show that these types of vague, summary memories reduce a person's ability to solve interpersonal problems. Why is this? To generate potential solutions to problems, a person needs to have access to the past in some detail. The past is their "database" from which to seek hints for how to deal with current problems. Overgeneral memories prevent a person from efficient use of his or her own "database." For example, if a person feels defeated or rejected, it would be helpful for her to have efficient access to specific times in the past when she has felt successful, loved, or respected. A categoric memory that only summarizes a number of occasions (e.g., "I used to go for walks with friends") is less useful than even one specific occasion (e.g., "I was out for a walk last month when I met Tim, and we met Sally and went back for coffee"). The specific event contains within it more "hints" for ways to solve current problems (there is "the walk," "Tim," "the coffee," and the possibility that these items would also cue other specific aspects of the event, such as the topics they talked about). So the specific memory contains within it several cues to help generate ideas about what action might be taken to escape from the feeling of defeat and rejection.

ENHANCING SPECIFIC MEMORIES

The research on overgeneral memory has implications for psychological treatment.

Should therapist and patient become stuck during therapy, it may help to know the possible reasons why such difficulties are occurring, and to practice detailed recollection of past events (e.g., starting by recalling relatively neutral events from the past week).

It is interesting to note how many psychological therapies include detailed rehearsal of each component of what led to occasions (between and within sessions) where suicidal urges or behavior occurred. And many therapists know that helping patients to call up vivid specific examples of reasons for living as opposed to generic categories is more helpful in therapy ("my son's pleasure when I read to him last night" as opposed to "my children").

When we first discovered the overgeneral memory phenomenon, we thought it might have implications for why some people become stuck in depression, while others seem to recover more quickly. In fact, a number of studies have now shown exactly this: that overgeneral memory, assessed near the beginning of an episode of depression, predicts how long the episode will last (Williams et al., 2007). Furthermore, in patients with a history of deliberate self-harm (DSH) over their lifetimes, those who have experienced childhood abuse are more likely to continue to attempt suicide, but even more so if they suffer from overgeneral memory (Sinclair, Crane, Hawton, & Williams, 2007). Finally if a person is overgeneral in memory during the late teenage years, he or she is more likely to become depressed in reaction to life stresses over the college years (Anderson, Goddard, & Powell, 2010; Gibbs & Rude, 2004; Stange, Hamlat, Hamilton, Abramson, & Allo, 2013; Sumner et al., 2011; Rawal & Rice, 2012).

When we later became interested in the mindfulness approach to preventing depression, we were interested in whether its emphasis on teaching participants to focus on moment-by-moment experience in a nonjudgmental way, and to recognize the tendency to avoid and instead to turn toward difficulties, would help people retrieve events in a more specific and less schematic way. In fact, an early study examining the impact of MBCT training in preventing relapse in depression showed that such training did indeed reduce the tendency toward overgeneral memory (Williams, Teasdale, Segal, & Soulsby, 2000); this finding has since been replicated (Heeren, Van Broeck, & Philippot, 2009). Having more specific memories after MBCT means that different possible solutions to difficult situations would suggest themselves (see "Enhancing Specific Memories," above). For instance, before mindfulness training, if a person's friend passed her in the street without seeing her, she might normally have come rapidly to the conclusion that this was just one more (typical) occasion when someone rejected her. Following training, she would be more likely to notice some other details about the event: that the traffic was busy, or that her friend was not wearing glasses, information that might suggest alternative explanations. Applying this sense of greater specificity to more situations is likely to weaken the sense of being trapped, as it will naturally reveal more possible ways to deal skillfully with problems in living

Rescue Factors

We have seen how attentional and memory processes may combine to affect the risk of suicidal feelings and behavior. However, we also noted, in the "defeated bird" analogy, that the longer-term prospects for the defeated animal depended upon whether it was rescued, that is, removed to a place of safety where recovery could take place. This suggested that there may be a third psychological process: the judgment by an individual about whether "rescue" is possible. What processes determine whether people believe that they themselves, other people, or circumstances will change for the better? How do people estimate the likelihood that something positive may happen involving their relationships, their jobs, their financial situations, and so on? To examine these questions more closely, we turned to the research on the psychology of judgment, and in particular to the domain of "prospective cognition."

Research on prospective cognition examines, for example, judgments about the risks of negative events such as getting cancer or getting burgled, and about the chance of positive events such as getting a promotion or winning the lottery. One conclusion of this research is that judgment about the future is partly made on the basis of a quick heuristic (rule of thumb), in this case, how fluently one is able to generate images of the scenario in question (Kahneman, 2012). It is unclear whether suicidal people are too fluent at thinking of negative future events that might happen, or not fluent enough at thinking of positive events.

In a study to examine this particular issue we matched suicidal patients (for age and educational level) with nondepressed hospital patients and a third group of people from the community (MacLeod, Rose, & Williams, 1993). Participants generated as many events as they could think of (even trivial events) that were likely to happen over (1) a day, (2) a week, (3) a month, (4) a year, and (5) 10 years. For each period, participants were given 30 seconds to come up with as many events as possible. The task was run through three times. On the first trial, participants were not given any instructions about whether the events to be generated were to be positive or negative. But on the second and third runs through (and in counterbalanced order across participants), they were told to generate *positive* events that might occur ("things you are looking forward to") or *negative* events that might occur ("things you are not looking forward to").

The results showed that suicidal patients were no more fluent in generating future negative events than the control groups. However, they were *less* fluent in coming up with possible future *positive* events. This suggests that the important difference between the suicidal and nonsuicidal participants was the relative lack of positive rescue factors for the suicidal group, rather than the excessive anticipation of negative things in the future. Further, the less fluent participants were in generating future positive possibilities, the more hopeless they were on Beck's Hopelessness Scale (Beck, Weissman, Lester, & Trexler, 1974), a well-known scale that predicts suicidal feelings in depression and how likely people are to commit suicide in the long term (Beck, Brown, Berchick, Stewart, & Steer, 1990). We concluded that hopelessness consists of an inability to imagine things that might happen in the future to "rescue" the situation.

One aspect of these results was particularly interesting for clinical approaches to hopelessness. Because the study required people to generate positive or negative items over several time periods (from 1 day to 10 years) it was possible to examine whether hopelessness mainly affected a person's long-term view of their future, or mainly affected a short-term view. The results showed that time interval made no difference (see the sidebar on p. 26).

ACCESSING A POSITIVE FUTURE

Those who have most difficulty constructing a positive long-term future for themselves are equally unlikely to be able to come up with something positive that might occur within the next 24 hours. This is important. When someone who comes to a therapist or mindfulness class is hopeless, it can seem that the feeling arises wholly from a sense that his or her whole life holds no promise, stretching into the far distance. One implication of this research is that it is okay, indeed important, to encourage people to see clearly how their mood might be affecting their sense of how the next few days will go, and that understanding the *near* future is as important as being drawn into focusing on larger issues of how the next few years will unfold.

Trapped and Hopeless: Self-Defeating Modes

This book takes us beyond the research we had done in the past about the associations between suicidal depression and these cognitive factors. The aim of our 10-year program of research was to see if these processes could be modified, and whether in particular mindfulness might help. We began to see that the ways people think about themselves when they are feeling depressed and hopeless can entrap them, so that their best attempts to rescue or fix their moods actually make things worse. The way we have come to understand this situation will be described in more detail later in the book, but here we give a general outline.

Think of the mind as having two modes of operation through which it processes information about the self, *conceptual* and *experiential* (see Chapter 4). These modes are shown in Figure 2.1 (Watkins, 2008; Watkins & Moulds, 2005; Williams, 2008). This rough model assumes that all input from the inner or outer world has first to be experienced through the senses. This input includes direct sensory experience of the external world—tasting, hearing, seeing, touching, and smelling—and also gut feelings (visceral sensations) and the sense of the body in space (proprioceptive sensations). People are taking this information in all the time, relatively automatically, and at the same time the mind is creating internally generated *concepts about* it. In each moment, the mind is labeling the input, elaborating it with associative memories, analyzing, judging, and comparing; it is planning and remembering and self-reflecting. While the conceptual system is enormously useful, it can sometimes create problems. This is particularly the case where people are in danger of *overthinking*.

We see overthinking in the way people react to their own emotions. Emotions such as sadness hardly ever come alone—there is the

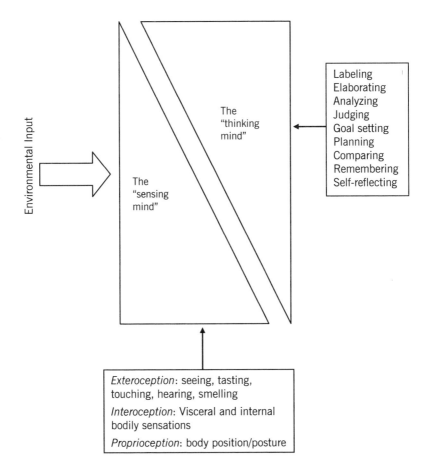

FIGURE 2.1. Two modes in which the mind operates: conceptual (language-based) processing versus sensory–perceptual processing. In every moment, we are receiving sights, sounds, tastes, smells, touch—stimuli from the external and internal world. But we generally ignore these stimuli in favor of spending most of our attention in conceptual mode. Based on Williams (2008).

primary feeling, then, hard on its heels, a secondary set of reactions. These secondary reactions are habitual attempts to make things better (e.g., an inner command to "snap out if it"), but they often make the feeling persist or even escalate. Primary emotions are signals that something is going right or wrong in life. As signals, they evolved to be temporary: to switch on when needed (e.g., when danger or loss threatens), and then switch off when the situation is past. A signal only "works" if it meshes accurately with the *actuality* of threats and losses, successes and surprises.

But humans have evolved the extraordinary ability to generate *ideas*. They can work "offline"—*recollect* events long gone, and *imagine* a future that has not yet happened. So the human mind and body has a new problem: it reacts not only to *real* dangers and losses, but also to secondary, self-generated *images* and *thoughts* of past or future dangers or losses. For responding to actual dangers, all animals have evolved freeze, flight, or fight mechanisms. These are hard-wired into the brain. But for humans these ancient parts of the brain sometimes do not distinguish between a real threat and an imagined or remembered situation. You cannot run fast enough to escape an *imagined* danger, yet the body gears up as if about to try. Most tragic of all, the mind reacts to its own emotions as if they were dangerous in themselves, and need to be gotten rid of. The result is that emotions, as experienced, are normally a mixture of the primary emotion and a secondary "reaction" to it, and it is difficult to tell where the primary emotion stops and the secondary reaction starts. The secondary reaction treats the emotion itself as a threat, and is driven to get rid of it.

The main ways in which people try to get rid of an emotion are either by suppressing it or by analyzing it. So if a person feels sad, the mind may immediately start to suppress the sadness or analyze "*Why* am I feeling sad?" Both suppression and analysis can tragically backfire and make things worse. *Suppression* of thoughts and feelings can make them more intrusive. (Try not thinking of a white bear for a minute. As Daniel Wegner, 1994, has pointed out, it's very difficult.) And *analysis* can involve endlessly raking over the past to understand "Why am I feeling like this, what does it mean about me, and where will it end?"

Self-Defeating Modes and Suicide Risk

We have seen that the ways in which people try to escape their own feelings—in particular through a misapplication of the conceptual mind—only makes things worse when the "ideas" generated by the conceptual mind exacerbate the original feeling. Compounded by biased attention to signals of defeat, wanting to escape but feeling trapped, and having no prospect of rescue, the result can be a sense of unbearable mental pain.

We may begin to see how all these processes contribute to suicidal behavior. Yet it remains true that many people experience mental pain and even suicidal thoughts from time to time, but they do not engage in actual suicidal behavior. This has led many to conclude that one can ignore such thoughts. Yet Louis Appleby's research in Manchester has found that such ideation is one of the clearest predictors of suicide in people with serious mental illness (Appleby, Dennehy, Thomas, Faragher, & Lewis, 1999). We need to know why it persists and keeps coming back.

We suggest in the next chapter that *differential activation* of suicidal ideation by different mood states may be a large part of the answer (cf. Teasdale, 1988, 1999). In the past of those who have been depressed, some will have experienced suicidal thoughts, and this pattern of thinking will have become associated with depressed mood *and any other moods or thoughts that were present at the time.* These additional moods may include anger, confusion, and frustration; the thoughts may include ideas such as "I am abandoned," "I am worthless," and "I am a burden." In the future, the recurrence of these other moods and/ or thoughts, even in the absence of depression, may be sufficient to trigger suicidal ideas. Now, of course, there are some people who have become suicidal without warning, the first time they were depressed— and this is tragically true of young men. But for most people seen in the clinic who are suicidal, there is a history in which the idea of death and suicide has become linked to certain key patterns of mood and cognition, with a different pattern for each person, and this pattern remains ready to be triggered by a recurrence of any one element of the pattern in the future.

Concluding Remarks

Searching for new and better ways to offer the alternative of life to those who seek our help is important, and we need a deeper understanding of what is going on. We offer the cry of pain ("arrested flight") as a framework for understanding the suicidal mind because we believe it offers a more comprehensive view of the problem than many alternatives, and because the concept of entrapment is readily translatable into terms that social and biological theories can also work with. Suicidal people are hardly ever certain that they want to die, but they certainly do not want to go on living in such pain . . . and our job is to help them find a way of living alongside the difficulties, making peace with despair, and giving them a chance to experience what it is like to come out on the other side of feeling so trapped.

CHAPTER 3

Why the Idea of Suicide
Won't Let Go

How could the triggering of such ancient self-defeating modes and their escalation into suicidal crisis be prevented? We know from research that there are a number of factors that increase the risk of suicidality: in most cases suicide occurs in the context of depression (Oquendo, Currier, & Mann, 2006), anxiety (Cougle, Keough, Riccardi, & Sachs-Ericsson, 2009), and hopelessness (Coryell & Young, 2005). Preventing recurrence of depression and related factors would thus go a long way toward preventing suicidality (Rihmer, 2001). However, only a proportion of those who get depressed become suicidal, and of those, only a proportion move from ideation to acting on their ideation. In order to specifically target suicidality, we would have to know more about the reasons why the suicidal mind state is brought on line again and again when some patients become depressed.

Reactivation of Depressive Thinking

Previous work on relapse in depression provided an important starting point for this endeavor. MBCT for relapse prevention had been developed based on a comprehensive new understanding of the mechanisms that are involved in the risk of recurrence of depression, and the processes that led to increases of this risk over time (Teasdale,

1999; Teasdale, Segal, & Williams, 1995). Two mechanisms were found to be of particular importance in this context. First of all, research had demonstrated that, in previously depressed patients, the negative thinking that was predominant during episodes of depression could be easily reactivated ("cognitive reactivity"). Experiments had shown that even subtle triggers such as small changes in mood could bring back, with great ferocity, beliefs that seem benign but are entrapping (Miranda & Persons, 1988)—for instance the beliefs "my self-worth depends totally on approval by others" or "I must succeed at *everything* or it means I am a failure" (see the sidebar below).

Importantly, research has demonstrated that the degree to which patients show such cognitive reactivity significantly predicts later relapse. That is, the more strongly patients responded to subtle changes in mood with reactivation of dysfunctional beliefs, the more likely they were to relapse (Segal et al., 2006). This seemed to be a central mechanism in relapse.

Second, there was a good understanding in the field of how particular forms of thinking could maintain negative mood. A large body of research had demonstrated that, when mood worsens, those who have been previously depressed often respond by repetitively thinking about the causes and consequences of their negative mood. Although such

LATENT MALADAPTIVE BELIEFS

Previous experiences of depression and other negative events may lead people to develop maladaptive beliefs that rigidly link self-worth with performance and approval from others:

"I cannot find happiness without being loved by another person."

"People who have the marks of success/good looks/fame/wealth are bound to be happier than people who do not."

"I should be happy all the time."

"Turning to someone else for help or advice is an admission of weakness."

Mood-related reactivation of such old beliefs means that people who have been depressed before are in danger of almost automatically engaging in negative thinking even during times when they are relatively well. All it needs is a small dip in mood and the cascade will start.

ruminative thinking starts as an attempt at closing the gap between current and desired states, it eventually serves an avoidant function, compromises people's ability to actively cope with their difficulties, and leads into self-perpetuating cycles of negative mood and thinking that paradoxically maintain negative mood (Nolen-Hoeksema, Wisco, & Lyubomirsky, 2008). Furthermore, there was the possibility that such a style of thinking might also have more long-lasting implications for the course of emotional problems. Cognitive accounts of vulnerability to recurrent depression had argued that as people repeatedly engaged in rumination, associations between mood and negative thinking were formed and reinforced, so that over time cognitive reactivity was likely to increase (Segal, Williams, Teasdale, & Gemar, 1996). When reactivity increases, so does the risk of recurrence with each new episode of depression, a process that is very much in line with the epidemiological observation of increasing risk of relapse with number of previous episodes.

Teasdale (1988) had used the term "differential activation" to refer to the fact that during previous experiences of depression, negative mood and other triggers acquired the potential to activate the negative thinking typical of depressive episodes. While they are in a normal mood, previously depressed people are similar in their thinking to those who have never been depressed. But once negative mood is present, it is likely to activate different responses in those who have previously been depressed. In our classes we sometimes use the Buddhist metaphor of the two arrows (described in the Sallatha Sutta) to explain this idea. In this metaphor, which illustrates the difference between pain and suffering, the first arrow refers to events that bring physical or emotional pain. Because not many things are under people's control, it is inevitable that they will be confronted with painful experiences. However, while the pain that comes with an actual experience (the first arrow) is unavoidable, there often is a reaction to the experience (the second arrow). What arises from this second arrow reflects the meaning given to the initial pain and the situation that caused it, and is influenced by a person's own temperament, what has happened to him or her in the past or recently, and his or her mood at the time the event occurs. This is what is meant by suffering: the pain that follows thinking, for example, "This should not have happened," "This is my fault," "This shows how inadequate I am," "This means things will never get better." In contrast to the first arrow, the degree to which the second arrow is fired and where it lands is controllable, or at least, trainable. What the research into the mechanisms underlying relapse in depression suggests that, in people with a history of recurrent depression, "first arrows" that inflicted mild emotional pain could cause significant suffering because of particular sets of learned beliefs and assumptions ("second arrows") that would lead people to attach a negative meaning to this emotional pain, and then respond to this meaning by repetitively thinking about its causes and consequences. MBCT for the prevention of relapse to depression had been designed to address exactly these mechanisms. Could such mechanisms be similarly relevant to recurrence of suicidality?

A Differential Activation Account of Suicidal Thinking

A first hint came from an analysis of relapse data from a previous trial of MBCT (Williams, Crane, Barnhofer, Van der Does, & Segal, 2006). This study allowed us to prospectively investigate how much each different symptom of depression tends to return when the syndrome recurs. The research followed participants over a longer period of time so we could see whether the particular symptoms people reported during their last episode of depression would also be part of their depression if they relapsed. It turned out that suicidality was the most consistent symptom, other than depressed mood and anhedonia, that is, loss of interest and pleasure, which is at the core of the definition of depression. Most of us tend to think of depression, when it returns again and

---

ASSESSING "WORST EVER" PAST SUICIDALITY

The finding that people who have been suicidal during past episodes of depression have a high risk of becoming suicidal again during later episodes of depression is clinically important. When assessing someone who is depressed, it is not enough to ask if he or she feels suicidal at the moment, but also how things have been at their worst time in the past. For we know now that as the depression deepens, if he or she has been suicidal in the past, such feelings are likely to recur.

again, as involving the same set of symptoms. But, surprisingly, most symptoms of depression show little or no consistency. For example, when depression returns someone who had eating problems in a previous episode may now not have them, and someone who did not have a sleep problem may now find he or she cannot sleep at all. But for suicidality the pattern is different. More than 80% of participants fell into the *same* category across different episodes—either being suicidal in both previous and subsequent episodes, or *not* being suicidal in both (see the sidebar on p. 34).

What Happens in Those at Risk of Suicide When Depression Recurs?

Chapter 2 described modes of self-defeat, sets of processes that we suspect are active in suicidality, brought about by a sense of "arrested flight" (similar to those suggested by Joiner, Rudd, & Rajab, 1997). Was it possible that these modes could be reactivated in those who had been suicidal during past episodes of depression, just as depressive thinking was reactivated in those who had been depressed in the past? Figure 3.1 shows how, if symptoms of depression (Figure 3.1a) occur together repeatedly, they form associations (Figure 3.1b). Some of these will be shared between people, but some will have features unique to each person.

It seemed crucial to us to understand more about what happens once depression and suicidal thinking have become linked. We were helped by a visit to Oxford University by a colleague from Leiden University who was studying reactivation of symptoms of depression. Van der Does had developed a way of assessing Teasdale's differential activation theory without having to ask previously depressed patients to undergo a possibly painful mood induction procedure. Using a similar procedure to that used by Nolen-Hoeksema to investigate rumination, Van Der Does was asking people to imagine that their mood was somewhat lower than normal, and then to indicate how much they found themselves experiencing a range of thoughts and feelings (using a standardized questionnaire, the LEIDS; Van der Does, 2002). He had not included suicidal items on the first version of this scale, but agreed to do so when he heard we were interested in this specific

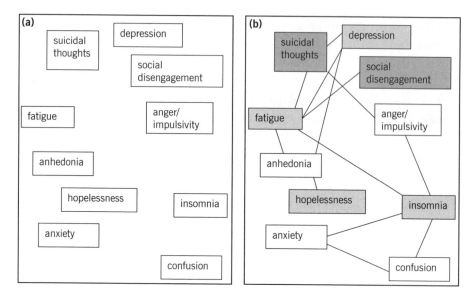

FIGURE 3.1. Associations between symptoms of depression in people with (b) and without (a) a history of depression.

issue. Both research teams began to use it to investigate how accessible such thoughts were to people even when they were not depressed. The research found that people (who we knew on the basis of other clinical assessments to have been suicidal during previous episodes of depression), endorsed the LEIDS items assessing hopelessness and suicidal ideation much more strongly than those who had a history of depression without suicidal ideation. In contrast, the two groups did not differ on other items such as those measuring aggression and harm avoidance (Williams, Van der Does, Barnhofer, Crane, & Segal, 2008). These studies provided us with further evidence that in those with a *history* of suicidal ideation or behavior, depressed mood more readily *reinstates* hopelessness and suicidal ideation.

One of the criticisms that can be made of the LEIDS procedure is that it is questionnaire-based and does not assess how sad people are feeling when they complete it. So, in a further step, we investigated whether these self-reports were related to how participants *actually* responded behaviorally when in a negative mood. In Chapter 2 we described research by MacLeod (MacLeod, Pankhania, Lee, & Mitchell, 1997) that showed that lack of fluency in generating positive future events is a driving force behind hopelessness. We took the same fluency task and gave it to a sample of people known to have been previously depressed and suicidal, before and after a mood induction in which negative mood was induced through playing sad music (Prokovief's "Russia under the Mongolian Yoke" at half speed) as background to reading sad statements. We found that participants' reports of how much they tended to respond to low mood with hopelessness and suicidality in the past significantly predicted reductions in positive future fluency following mood induction. This was remarkable to witness: when mood was okay, everyone could generate positive things they were looking forward to in the future. Now, only 10 minutes later, after a simple mood induction that shifted mood just a few points on a scale, people with a history of hopelessness now found it much more difficult to do so. This finding confirmed for us that what people had reported was actually reflected in their thinking at the very time their mood changed, and provided first insight into the reactivation of a suicidal mode of thinking.

> A small downward shift in sad mood has a subtle but critical impact on those who have been suicidal and hopeless in the past: it blocks the mind's access to positive events in the future (see Williams, Van der Does, Barnhofer, Crane, & Segal, 2008).

Hopelessness about the future reflects only one of the different facets of the cry of pain: the sense of being trapped. Even if a person could not come up with future positive experiences, one might think that he or she would at least be able to struggle through with his or her current issues and problems. Not so. Around the same time we had embarked on a laboratory study that focused on mood-related changes on another aspect of cognitive functioning that we already knew was of central importance in suicidality: the ability to solve social problems.

When as a clinician or therapist or friend, you meet someone who has lost a loved one to suicide, they often are not surprised that their loved one felt depressed, or even suicidal. Anyone can understand loneliness, despair, and a sense of hopelessness when things go wrong. But what family and friends say more often are things like, "Why now?", "Why didn't they call?", "She seemed fine when I saw her last week?", "Why didn't he do something, *anything*, but this?"

Why do suicidal people determine that suicide is their only recourse? Our previous research, and that of many others, had revealed part of the answer. When someone feels hopeless and despairing, suicide seems the only option because other options seem invisible, impossible, or out of reach. This is why people feel totally defeated and trapped until the absence of relief from the mental pain becomes unbearable (Pollock & Williams, 1998).

> After a suicide, many urgent questions arise among close family and friends: "Why now?", "Why didn't he call?", "Why didn't she do something, *anything*, but this?" It is a tragic fact that when someone feels hopeless and despairing, suicide seems the only option because other options just don't seem available.

We set out to see whether depressed patients who were now well carry with them a hidden sign of their history of suicidal feelings and behavior. We knew that many people who become seriously depressed never feel suicidal despite their suffering. Others do. When mood is back to normal, there is no apparent difference in problem-solving abilities between those who have been depressed in the past and those who have never been depressed—and no difference between those who have been depressed with or without a history of suicidal feelings and behavior.

But what would happen if all these different people came into the laboratory one by one, and listened for 10 minutes to the sad music and read sad statements. We assessed their social problem solving using scenarios that described commonly experienced personal problems, for example, "You have moved into a new neighborhood and don't know anyone" or "You are having trouble with your supervisor." Each scenario ended with positive conclusions: "In the end you have many friends" or "You end up getting on well with your supervisor." Their task was simple: to describe how they would go about solving the problem. We assessed how effective the solutions were before and after the 10-minute negative mood induction.

As expected, the three groups (never depressed, depressed without suicidal history, and depressed with a suicidal history) did not differ in social problem-solving ability before the mood induction, and all three groups showed comparable changes in mood following the Prokofiev. Once again, the results after the mood challenge were striking. Participants with a history of depression and also suicidality showed significantly larger deteriorations in problem-solving ability following the induction than *either* previously depressed participants without a history of suicidality *or* never-depressed participants (Williams, Barnhofer, Crane, & Beck, 2005). Only 10 minutes of a slightly sad mood had revealed a hidden vulnerability: suddenly these participants who had been fine a little while ago were now suffering a sort of solution blindness. Talking afterward they were glad to reflect with us on how similar this is to what happens in everyday life. They can be going along on firm ground, then something happens to tip their mood slightly and they find themselves struggling against slipping into quicksand: nothing comes to mind that might help, and everything that does come to mind is irrelevant.

> Altogether the findings from these studies clearly supported the idea that there were particular patterns of mind (hopelessness, suicidal thoughts, and deficits in social problem solving) that were habitual and automatic reactions for some. In people who have been suicidal in the past, a small increase in negative mood *now* directly activates the very processes that were present during *past* suicidal crises. But it is not clear to the person that this is the past—everything *now* feels hopeless and pointless.

Once suicidal thinking is reactivated, what determines whether it escalates? It was plausible, of course, to assume that the mechanisms we knew were involved in the maintenance of negative mood and thinking in depression in general would be relevant here too. Rumination about the causes and consequences of the crisis, attempts to suppress negative thoughts and to avoid their toxic downstream effects on feelings and impulses are common responses to negative mood that paradoxically maintain the mood, and that are likely to be present in suicidal depression too. In fact, given the aversiveness of the suicidal mind state, it was conceivable that previously suicidal patients would be even more likely to engage in deliberate self-harm as an attempt to control suicidal thoughts and impulses. From our previous research (see Chapter 2) we knew that depressed patients had pronounced deficits in remembering autobiographical events and tended to relate to their past by thinking about whole classes or categories of events rather than retrieving particular instances (Williams et al., 2007). As we described in Chapter 2, when given cue words such as "happy," they would be likely to come up with responses such as "Whenever I am with friends," rather than recalling an occasion relating to a particular day and place. This overgenerality makes ruminative tendencies more likely, undermines people's ability to solve social problems (Pollock & Williams, 2001), and seemed particularly pronounced in people with suicidal depression, suggesting that these people might experience even more difficulties disengaging from negative ruminative thinking (Pollock & Williams, 1998). When we looked at the data from our experiment on mood induction and problem solving, we noticed that people in the group with a history of suicidality differed from one another in how overgeneral their memory was. This allowed us to examine if the overgeneral memory made a difference in the impact of mood on problem solving. It made a large difference. Those who had difficulty being specific in their memory for the past were twice as impaired in their problem solving after the sad music as those with specific memories.

Altogether, this line of research suggested that the differential activation mechanisms that we knew were relevant in relapse to depression in general were also involved in relapse to suicidality. If you have been depressed in the past, negative patterns of mind lie ready and waiting to be reactivated. If you have *also* been suicidal, then there are additional patterns of mind lying ready when sad mood strikes: hopelessness, an inability to see any positive future, and an inability to see a way out of current problems. It was differential activation theory that had informed the rationale for MBCT for prevention of depression. We became more confident that MBCT might have promise as an approach to the problem of suicidal depression as well.

Beyond Cognitive Reactivation: The Characteristics of Suicidal Thinking

Would this understanding of the suicidal mind be enough to proceed: Would it allow for a sufficiently nuanced and effective approach? We conducted an exploratory trial in which previously suicidal patients were allocated either to receive a slightly modified version of MBCT immediately, or to wait until the end of the treatment phase. We tested participants before and after this phase. Results were positive. In addition to being feasible and acceptable for people with a history of suicidal depression, our data, collected through interviews, question- naires, and experimental tasks, suggested that participants had clearly profited from the approach. It seemed that MBCT could feasibly be transferred to people with suicidal depression.

However, it turned out that there was some important information that we had missed. This became apparent when our colleagues Emily Holmes and Catherine Crane interviewed a number of participants from our trial to investigate suicidal imagery. In a large number of previous studies, Holmes and colleagues had investigated the effect of imagery in emotional disorders, and had convincingly demonstrated that the emotional impact of images was potentially much stronger than the impact of verbal thinking (Holmes & Mathews, 2005). Partic- ularly in trauma-related disorders (Ehlers & Clark, 2000), but also in depression and other disorders (Brewin, Gregory, Lipton, & Burgess, 2010), intrusive images were known to be a common occurrence and to be experienced by people as highly distressing. Furthermore, there was good evidence showing that mental imagery could increase the probability of future behavior such as voting in elections (e.g., Libby, Shaeffer, Eibach, & Slemmer, 2007). We had to confront a worrying possibility. If imagery made the behavior that was being imagined more likely to be actually enacted, then it might be the case that some people had frequent images of killing themselves that would make the suicidal act more likely. Up to that point, the role of imagery in sui- cidal crises had not been explored in much detail in suicidal patients. We thought we had assessed our participants thoroughly, asking them about their suicidal thoughts and whether they found plans to commit suicide going through their minds.

Emily Holmes, and her colleague Ann Hackmann, were very experienced in assessing patients suffering from posttraumatic stress disorder (PTSD), and they had shown that you have to ask specific questions about the actual sensory details of imagery (e.g., in a PTSD flashback) to get the full picture. These images can be hard to admit to, and can bring back intense and difficult feelings, so it is no won- der that both patients and clinicians may shy away from investigating them. In order to investigate further, Emily Holmes teamed up with Catherine Crane to conduct interviews with participants in our first classes (all of whom had been depressed and suicidal in the past) and asked them a structured series of questions about the times when they were most despairing. What they found was surprising. All of the participants reported experiencing extensive and intrusive images, most often scenarios where they saw themselves acting out their suicidal ideas, often in disturbing detail. Some had sensory images of being dead or of locations that would provide the opportunity for suicide (Holmes, Crane, Fennell, & Williams, 2007). What disturbed us was how much we had missed. We had not asked the right questions in the right way. Linking up with the "flashbacks" that are a common and disturbing occurrence in victims of trauma, we called this phenomenon "flashforwards." Flashforwards are both common and underreported; yet they may be one of the most powerful drivers of the unbearable mental pain that those who come to us for help are suffering.

It doesn't stop there. Flashbacks play an important role in the maintenance of PTSD *not* because of their occurrence per se, but because of the way in which people react to them (Ehlers & Clark, 2000). Flashbacks are bad enough, but in addition, there is a second arrow: the flashbacks are interpreted as signs of impending danger (e.g., "It's going to happen again," "I'm going mad"), leading to steps aimed at wanting to keep the worst from happening. These often take the form of avoidance and suppression, and therefore prevent emotional processing and risk keeping initial fears and concerns alive. Similarly, the flashforwards our participants reported seemed to play an important role in the development of suicidal feelings: the more preoccupied people reported to have been with the images, and the more real the images had seemed to them at the time, the more severe their suicidal feelings had been. At the same time, however, it turned out that while all participants had experienced the images as distressing, many participants also reported soothing or calming effects. This latter finding was unpredicted, and therefore had to be interpreted cautiously. However, in a second study conducted with a more heterogeneous group of participants, similar results emerged. Furthermore, in this second study, conducted by Catherine Crane and colleagues (Crane, Shah, Barnhofer, & Holmes, 2012), participants who had rated their imagery as more soothing had experienced higher levels of suicidal ideation, suggesting that positive reactions to the images went together with a higher risk of acting on suicidal ideation. Given the detrimental effects suggested by these findings, not having explicitly addressed the effect of suicidal imagery in our classes was an omission that deeply concerned us. It clearly seemed important to better understand it.

What was of even more concern to us, though, was that participants had made little reference to suicidal imagery not only in our assessment interviews, but also in our MBCT classes, despite the fact that learning to approach what is difficult was an important and integral aspect of the program. Perhaps they preferred not to answer and risk reactivating these memories and images. This was a stark reminder of the emotional perturbation that was involved in suicidal crises. We now had to acknowledge that the emotional turmoil involved in those at risk of suicide was in many ways different from what individuals experienced in depression and anxiety. Orbach and colleagues (Orbach, Mikulincer, Sirota, & Gilboa-Schechtman, 2003; Orbach, Mikulincer, Gilboa-Schechtman, & Sirotas, 2003) had conducted work to elucidate the complexities of this experience.

Their work was based in part on early work by Shneidman (1985), who had coined the term "psychache," which he suggested arises when the individual feels that essential needs, such as the need for belonging, to have control, to protect one's self-image, to avoid shame, or to feel secure, are significantly thwarted or frustrated. This supposition was similar to that of interpersonal theories that highlighted the role of thwarted belongingness and perceived burdensomeness in suicidal ideation (Van Orden et al., 2010). Shneidman (1985) had suggested in his description that frustration of these needs would bring up a range of negative emotions (guilt, shame, defeat, humiliation, disgrace, grief, and hopelessness), which combined together would turn into a generalized experience of unbearable mental pain. Orbach and colleagues had suggested several defining characteristics of this experience, including a sense of irreversibility, of loss of control, and strong emotional responses such as emotional flooding and freezing, difficulties integrating changes in self-identity, confusion, social distancing, and loss of personal meaning. Mental pain, Orbach and colleagues asserted, represented an experiential entity in its own right, which, if it reached high intensity and individuals lost hope for change, would crucially drive suicidal behavior.

Consistent with this was evidence from another line of research. In a number of studies participants with increased sensitivity to anxiety (fear of fear) were found to be at an increased risk for suicidality. In particular, this research had highlighted the role of cognitive components of anxiety sensitivity, fear of loss of control or emotional intensity, reflected, for example, in statements such as "It is important for me to stay in control of my emotions" and "When I am nervous, I worry that I am mentally ill." In depressed patients, the presence of panic attacks, which are usually associated with strong anxiety sensitivity, was found to significantly predict suicide attempts (Katz, Yaseen, Mojtabai, Cohen, & Galynker, 2011). Similarly, in patients suffering from panic disorder, anxiety sensitivity was demonstrated to be an even stronger predictor of suicidal ideation than depressive symptoms (Schmidt, Woolaway-Bickel, & Bates, 2001). Other research showed relations between fear of loss of control and emotional intensity and suicidality in large outpatient samples.

Clearly these findings suggested that, in line with the finding that suicidal imagery could have both distressing and calming effects, those with the highest levels of fear of losing control and emotional intensity were at increased risk for suicide.

> Once mental pain is present, those with increased sensitivity for loss of control and emotional intensity are in greatest danger of resorting to images, thoughts, and actual suicide attempts as ways of freeing themselves from such pain.

While it was conceivable that such an idealized view of death as an escape from suffering may have little bearing on actual behavior initially, it was possible that the link might grow stronger over time and with repeated exposure to suicidality. Thomas Joiner and colleagues (Van Orden et al., 2010) had suggested that repeated exposure to suicidal crises means that people habituate. They become less fearful about negative effects, such as harming themselves. At the same time, more positive experiences (such as the relief of thinking about, imagining, or acting on what seems like a viable solution—harming or killing themselves) are likely to increase over time. Consistent with this supposition, research has shown that people with more previous episodes of depression feel more soothed and calmed following their most recent episode of self-harm (Gordon et al., 2010). It seemed that the fact that suicidal imagery could have both distressing and calming effects provided a window on a very similar dynamic.

Implications for a Mindfulness Approach
to Preventing Suicidal Crises

These findings had clear implications for our therapeutic approach. They stressed the importance of teaching people at risk of suicide how to relate to thoughts and images of suicide, and the accompanying mental pain, in a way that allowed them to hold this experience in awareness without resorting to the soothing escape these thoughts and images implied.

While we had taught in our classes that negative depressive thinking could, and needed to, be addressed with gentleness and openness, the images of suicide and flashforwards were so distressing and threatening that it seemed that the same gentle way of relating to thoughts could not apply to them. What we had learned from research clearly told us that it was necessary to invite participants to bring into the classes even the most distressing images of suicide. We had to explicitly raise the points that these were common occurrences in suicidal depression, and that these images could and needed to be addressed in very much the same way as other aspects of depressive thinking. We also had to raise the point that suicidal thinking could escalate quickly. In themselves, intrusive images could evoke strong emotional responses. It was not hard to imagine how feeling ashamed and out of control of the images, along with attempts to suppress and avoid them, might lead to an escalation into crisis much more quickly than the negative thinking commonly present in depression.

We saw more clearly now why people who were highly sensitive to anxiety were particularly vulnerable for developing suicidal behavior. And finally, we were even more aware of the importance of acknowledging the immense painfulness of suicidal images and thoughts. These were important points to be addressed in our classes. Just as we describe the territory of depression in MBCT, we would have to describe the territory of suicidality, even if going there seemed to be a more difficult journey. These are themes that we will return to in detail in Chapters 7–14, for these new understandings should affect our approach to anyone of us who offers help to those suffering from mental pain, however caused.

In the end, while we had thought suicidal depression contained two elements (the first arrow of the pain of a negative event, and the second arrow of suffering engendered by the meaning attached to that event), it seemed that for suicidal depression we had to elaborate the picture. In suicidal crises, people needed to be prepared for a third element—a third arrow: a strong and compelling sense of *urgency* following from that meaning, a sense *of having to do something* about the pain, *right now, immediately,* because otherwise it would be overwhelming, there would be an unbearable loss of control. We had to prepare participants not only for the fact that, just like other aspects of depressive thinking, suicidal thinking could be reactivated easily, but that it might come in shapes very different from other depressive thinking. In particular suicidal sensory imagery, flashforwards, may arise, and if they do they will plunge clients right into strong and seemingly unbearable mental pain.

> In suicidal crises, there is a third element—a third arrow. It is a strong and compelling sense of *urgency* to take action, a sense *of having to do something* about the pain *right now.*

Concluding Remarks

We had to remind participants that this pain was likely to come with a strong impulse of wanting to escape, wanting to do something about the pain. Yet, just as with other painful experiences, avoidance or suppression, although often helpful in the short term, were likely to lead into further problems. And clearly, this information needed to be conveyed in a balanced approach. In the turmoil of suicidal crises, the decision to distract themselves or avoid, might in some cases have been a lifesaving response. But from a longer-term perspective, we had to help participants find acceptant ways of dealing with even the most difficult of experiences. MBCT contained all the necessary ingredients to address this problem, but we would have to adjust the way they were taught and presented. Furthermore, these novel elements needed to be present from the first preclass interview, in our approach to people, in the way we talked to and "assessed" their willingness to participate in mindfulness.

CHAPTER 4

How Could Mindfulness Help?

Doing and Being

The insights from our own and other clinical researchers' discoveries suggested that MBCT contained all the necessary ingredients to address the problems we were seeing in our suicidal patients. Yes, there would need to be changes in exactly how these elements were offered, and in what was emphasized, and we will describe these changes in more detail in later chapters. But from early on, we were confident that MBCT could help sufferers, for three reasons.

First, Annette Beautrais and her colleagues (Beautrais et al., 1996) had found that depression was one of the most important preexisting conditions for suicidal behavior. One way of expressing this dependence is to use a statistic called the population attributable ratio (PAR). The PAR is the proportion of a population whose illness or syndrome is attributable to another factor (e.g., the proportion of lung cancer attributable to smoking is over 90%, meaning that one could save over 90% of lung cancers if no one smoked). Beautrais showed that the PAR for depression in serious suicidal behavior was 80%. This implies that if we could eliminate depression from the world, we would save 80% of suicidal behavior. Although no one expects to remove depression completely, of course, our previous research had found that MBCT did reduce the risk of depression in the most recurrent patients. Even if we did not address suicidal behavior itself, reducing the risk of its most important precursor was vitally important.

A second reassurance for using mindfulness to help those who were suicidal was that our colleague Linehan had used mindfulness practices as one of the central elements of her DBT for people suffering from borderline personality disorder (Linehan, 1993). Such sufferers experience frequent urges to harm themselves, sometimes with and sometimes without suicidal intent, and often wind up in the hospital or seeking help from family or friends after burning or cutting themselves, or taking overdoses of prescribed or nonprescribed medication. As we mentioned in Chapter 2, DBT combines individual therapy in which acts or urges to self-harm are always prioritized, with group skills training sessions. In the group sessions, people learn emotional self-regulation, distress tolerance, and interpersonal effectiveness, as well as participating in a specific module on mindfulness skills. Many patients report that the mindfulness skills they learn are the most important element in the whole program.

A final reassurance was that our previous research had found that mindfulness could help make a difference to one of the major processes in the buildup of suicidal behavior: the collapse of alternative ways of coping with difficulties. Such impairment in finding ways to cope with everyday problems can be the straw that breaks the camel's back. In the midst of a crisis, the inability to *see* a way through makes a person feel that there actually *is* no way through. Our research had found two things that were important to us: First, that such "solution blindness" is integrally linked with the way people remember events from their past. If they are overgeneral and overabstract in remembering events from the past, this significantly undermines their ability to come up with solutions to problems right now. Second, we had found that MBCT makes such autobiographical memory more specific, thus alleviating one of the critical vulnerability factors. It led to the hope that, even if people became depressed again after MBCT, perhaps they might be able to feel sad—even deeply sad—but without losing hope for the future. The hope was that they might be less likely to become suicidal again because they would be less likely to be trapped by constant brooding and self-analyzing, and thereby retain a sense that life might work out, and that it was worth staying alive to see it.

But how does MBCT bring about such changes? This is not just an academic question, but one with direct practical relevance that is often

asked by people who come to us seeking help. Here is what a mindfulness teacher often hears:

> "Will this help me? *Can* this help me?"
> "I've tried everything, and a friend said I should try this, but I
>   can't see how meditating 6 times a week will help. Can you
>   explain?"
> "I want to believe this will work, but someone told me that in
>   MBCT we don't talk about our problems. My life's been hor-
>   rible, how on earth can anything help that doesn't discuss my
>   problems and help me resolve them?"

So, How Does Mindfulness Help?

Critical to personal change is that a person is able to take a wider
perspective on his or her own thoughts, feelings, and impulses (captured in the phrase *metacognitive awareness*). "Metacognitive awareness" means the capacity to *experience* cognitions (thoughts, images,
assumptions, attitudes, beliefs) as events in the mind, learned mental
habits, rather than as a reflection of objective truth, or an integral
part of "me." Note that "experience" is printed in italics. This emphasizes the fact that metacognitive awareness is not purely intellectual or
theoretical, but also felt in the heart and in the gut: it is a whole-person
experience, not merely an idea. As this quality develops, people realize that it is not necessary to take their thoughts so personally, believe
them so absolutely, or do what they say. Thus choices in how best to
respond open up.

Metacognitive awareness allows a person to de-center from old
habits of thinking and feeling, to step back and see thoughts and feelings for what they are: transient mind and mood states. This is a bit like
standing beside a complex piece of machinery, observing with interest
how it works, what connects to what, what follows from what, without
getting so close there is a danger of being injured by the moving parts.
This is different from suppression or avoidance, on the one hand, and
overattachment to goals and ideals, on the other, because it is consciously done rather than being an automatic kneejerk reaction, and

because it has a quality of kindliness ("Ah, here is sadness—this is what sadness is like") and recognition ("Here's my self-critical thinking on the loose again"). Taking the treatment of depression as a paradigm case, research has shown how changes in the ability to de-center in this way underlie the potency of the best-known evidence-based therapy for depression (cognitive therapy) as well as of MBCT (Teasdale et al., 2002; Beiling et al., 2012).

What are the barriers to metacognitive awareness? Chief among them is the tendency to become entangled in thinking. As we've seen, thinking and analysis are very powerful in helping people make sense of the world. They allow people to go beyond the direct evidence of their senses to do counterfactual reasoning ("What if such and such had happened?"), to make inferences (if you hear that "Mary dropped a glass" and "John went to fetch a broom," then you infer that "A glass got broken"), and to build mental models of the situation that can help in solving the problem and suggesting what action might be taken next (checking that there is no broken glass left) (Teasdale et al., 1995).

The inner world such representations can create, in which humans differ from other animals in being able to retrieve and think about a past long gone, or to imagine and then elaborate a future not yet born, is an extraordinary evolutionary inheritance. It achieves so much, so we do not see its darker side—which may become clear only when analytic thinking volunteers for tasks for which it is the wrong tool. Much of our day-to-day problem solving involves a particular form of processing—*discrepancy-based processing*—wherein the use of such inner language easily entangles rather than liberates. "Discrepancy-based processing" refers to a focus on the mismatch (or discrepancy) between things as they are (including me as a person, and my mood and state of mind) and things as I *want* them to be, or think they *should* be. The short-hand for such discrepancy-based thinking is the "doing" mode of mind.

It is not inner language per se that is the problem so much as the fact that the doing mode often defaults to using inner language and analytic thinking as the sole "currency" of cognition in relation to our goals (that we are seeking to move toward) and antigoals (that we are seeking to avoid or escape). That is, humans have a tendency to try to *think* themselves out of unsatisfactory situations. As we shall see, in everyday life, this capacity is immensely useful. It allows us to define problems, to generate alternative potential solutions, to try them out, to check on progress ("discrepancy monitoring"), to evaluate the effectiveness of the solution we have attempted and, if necessary, to rethink and try again. But when these same strategies are applied to feelings, or to sense of self, they may backfire.

The doing mode has become hard wired into the brain during evolution. An animal moving across its territory, or jumping from one branch to another, needs to have a brain that can compute the gap between its current position and the place it wants to be (e.g., the opposite side of the terrain, or the next branch), and the movement needed to close the gap between them. Then it initiates the action of moving, monitoring the gap, repeatedly checking progress toward the goal until the terrain or branch is safely reached, after which doing mode can stop for that task; the goal is achieved.

So the doing mode is a vital aspect of our lives and normally works fluently and well for external problems (e.g., taking a package to the post office on the way to work). Why so? *Because the checking mechanism (monitoring the gap between where I am and where I want to be) does not itself affect the external circumstances.* That is, checking how far it is to the post office does not affect the actual distance left to travel.

But what happens when the problem is with our moods? In this case, the "gap" that needs to be closed is not a gap between where we are now and a desired destination, but between the mood that we find ourselves in and the mood we want to be in. This is the "mismatch" that has to be resolved. It is natural for us to believe that discrepancy-based, doing mode might help us solve this emotional problem. The goal is clear: to escape or avoid unhappiness, on the one hand, and to achieve happiness on the other, monitoring how we are getting on all the while. If you can think of a quick way of dealing with the mood (e.g., take a break, or go see a friend), there is no problem. But sometimes such practical tips don't come to mind, and we continue to focus on the mismatch itself. Such constant monitoring of how we fare against the standards of happiness we have set for ourselves turns out to be unhelpful. The doing mode—so useful for solving problems—now becomes *driven*-doing. Expressed in words, discrepancy-based processing can be hard to understand, so the sidebar on p. 52 offers you a small exercise to try.

DOING → DRIVEN-DOING:
A SMALL PERSONAL EXPERIMENT

We can illustrate the operation of how doing mode can tip into driven-doing in the following way.

Imagine you were feeling tired right now.

Perhaps take a moment to tune in to any sense of actual fatigue that's around for you, right now.

When you are ready, try this experiment:

Try slowly saying these phrases to yourself: "I wish I didn't feel like this"; "I don't want to feel like this"; "I wish I felt different"; "What will happen if it goes on?"

Allow these thoughts to swirl around, allowing the one that feels most relevant to you to remain for longer: "I wish I didn't feel like this"; "I don't want to feel like this"; "I wish I felt different"; "What will happen if it goes on?"

Now how do you feel? Many people say that just wishing they felt less tired makes them *more* tired. In Chapter 2 (see Figure 2.1), we drew a distinction between moment-by-moment sensory experience and thinking *about* the experience (using concepts and analysis). Discrepancy-based processing uses concepts to keep the mismatch in mind, and you may have just felt the result of such conceptual processing in the tiredness experiment.

We need to see clearly what is going on here. Why is it that many people feel more tired when they concentrate on how tired they feel and on the desire to feel different? The increased fatigue is the effect of the doing mode setting up the goal of *feeling more awake or energetic*, and the antigoal (to be avoided) of *feeling worse*. When you think in this way, you hold in mind the mismatch—so you end up not only with the fatigue you started with, but with the added sense of dissatisfaction, negativity, and tiredness from the prospect of having to do something about it. The result is that the gap between how you feel and how you want to feel is widening rather than closing. An everyday example of a similar process is when you can't sleep in the middle of the night: you toss and turn, wishing you could sleep, and getting even more tense as a result.

Now let us turn to why the same thing happens for negative mood. Two factors contribute to this escalation. First, as we've seen, the sense of a "mismatch" creates its own negative mood. Usually, such a slight increase in negative mood motivates you to take action. But with a mismatch between a mood (such as anxiety, anger, or unhappiness) and how you want to feel, the negativity from the mismatch itself can too easily (and without our noticing) mix with the original mood to make things worse. You were unhappy. The perception of the mismatch has made you even less happy.

The second reason why using the doing mode of mind can become "driven-doing" is that the "matching" process uses ideas and thoughts, and these—being abstract—are very likely to create new trains of thought: "I wish I didn't feel this bad when I need to be in top form. Why is this happening to me? Why do I always feel this way?" We are soon trapped in overthinking and, as Watkins has pointed out, move far away from the "how" of what would be the best way to help ourselves (Watkins, 2008).

> When the doing mode is used to fix your mood or your sense of "self" it can easily become *driven-doing*. In the driven-doing mode of mind, you feel you just cannot disengage from the goal of trying to get what you want (feeling better) or get rid of what you don't want (feeling despair).

Driven-doing mode of mind brings with it a feeling of being stuck. You may feel you just cannot let go of trying to get what you want or to get rid of what you don't want because your worsening mood makes the gap between current and desired state bigger. As Segal et al. (2013) explain, our natural drive for happiness creates patterns of thinking, feeling, and behavior that are unhelpful, because they simply circle round and round without producing a resolution. Many research studies find that attempts to "problem-solve" using ruminative/analytic processing actually *reduce* problem solving and maintain depression (Segal et al., 2013, p. 178).

Feeling a Stranger to Ourselves

We have pointed to how much humans use thinking—the medium of imagery and thought—as the basis for problem solving for most daily activities. The danger in this method of living is that the world can come to be seen "secondhand" through these ideas, thoughts, and images. Particularly at times of high emotion and distress, you see through the lens of your preexisting schemas, rather than with an unbiased awareness of things as they really are, right now. Priority is given to *thinking about* the world. Direct, sensory experience *of* the world fades from awareness. When sensory experience is ignored or taken for granted, you eventually work from secondhand ideas *about* what things look, taste, hear, smell, or feel like rather than noticing how things actually are. Similarly, if you spend a great deal of time thinking about yourself in doing (conceptual) mode rather than directly *experiencing*, you begin to feel a separation between different aspects of yourself. For many of our patients this separation has become really intense. They do not like the "self" that is created by their overthinking, they have begun to fantasize about escaping from it. You may even hear them saying "I cannot live with myself."

Shifting Modes of Mind

We have seen that, as a result of doing mode volunteering for a job it cannot do then tipping into driven-doing, the tendency for suicidal people to become entangled in thinking intensifies their despair and produces a state in which they simply cannot bear the pain of feeling this way any longer and will do anything to bring it to an end. How, then, do we teach participants in an MBCT class to recognize which mode they are in and, if they choose, to switch to an alternative mode?

The simple answer is that MBCT cultivates decentering by teaching mainly one thing: to bring attention to the body. It prioritizes the realm of sensation. Mindfulness uses the body as foundational, as a portal to an alternative way of knowing the self and the world (see the sidebar on pp. 55–56). Of course, in practice, mindfulness turns out to be more difficult than that. For the rest of this chapter, though, consider as an overriding theme the notion of turning attention to the body and sensation.

The challenge of paying sustained attention to the body arises from the driven-doing mode of mind always reasserting itself, in a variety of guises. Try focusing on any part of your body for a few moments,

THE BUDDHIST BACKGROUND:
THE BODY AS FOUNDATIONAL FOR MINDFULNESS

Those readers who are interested in the foundational Buddhist tradition from which mindfulness comes will recognize the emphasis on embodiment as consistent with the teaching that the body is the first foundation of (or "the first way of establishing") mindfulness.

We are grateful to our colleague, the Buddhist scholar and meditation teacher John Peacock, for pointing us to several of the (many) places where the earliest Buddhist writings sees the body as vitally important. The largest proportion of the Satipatthana Sutta (Discourse on the Four Ways of Founding Mindfulness) is devoted to mindfulness of the body. On the evidence of this sutta and many others, the teachings assert that we are dangerously estranged from our bodies. "Being at home in the body" requires a degree of awareness, which in its quality and fullness, calls for the kind of cultivation practices outlined in the Satipatthana Sutta.

The teachings record the Buddha as stating that he realized awakening, "within his six foot-body." Living in this way requires that a person be grounded right here, where life is unfolding moment by moment: *in the body* "with its perceptions and conceptions," that is, *in feelings, mind, mental qualities, and phenomena.* The primary locus for the unfolding of life is thus based on bodily experience. The teachings call this a "diligent" rather than a "negligent" way of living: "The diligent do not die, those who are negligent are as the dead." "Diligence" is here a synonym for that which leads to the awakened way of life.

In the Anguttara Nikaya (The Numerical Discourse of the Buddha) it says, even more strongly, that one who has not established mindfulness of the body will not reach an awakened way of living—the equivalent of having no mindfulness at all.

> Monks they partake not of the Deathless [synonym for the awakened state] who partake not of mindfulness centred on the body. (Anguttara Nikaya. I.21.47)

The teachings caution us to cease being hijacked every time some object that is "pleasing, desirable, charming, agreeable and enticing" comes in front of us. Notice that these texts do not harangue us about the "sins of the flesh" which is just another way of invoking aversion, hostility and delusion, but by encouraging us to pay attention to our "natural habitat." He says, "live within your native domain" and it is by living in this native domain that we are given the ability to "choose."

(continued)

> Of course, it is no accident that MBSR/MBCT's practice of prioritizing the body agrees with traditional teaching, for mindfulness as it is taught in the West has always sought to remain faithful to the founding traditions in their most universal application, without seeking to restrict participants to a particular faith or philosophy. The philosophy underlying the modern Western practice of mindfulness suggests that perceiving the external or internal world *directly*, rather than indirectly through the medium of the thinking mind's concepts, judgment, analysis, and comparison, is available to anyone who commits to doing the mental training that is required to cultivate this clear sensing of the body moment by moment.

and you may soon find that you start thinking about something else, for instance, something you meant to do and have forgotten, something that happened yesterday or last week—or sometimes many months or even years ago. The task of the doing mode is to find unfinished business and bring it to mind. This it will do again and again and again.

> MBCT prioritizes the realm of *sensation*. It uses the body as foundational, a portal to an alternative way of knowing the self and the world.

If we are to help those for whom the "unfinished business" involves dealing with a great deal of trauma and hardship from the past, or trying to find ways to avoid an imagined future that is too hard to bear, we need to do more than say that driven-doing mode is the problem and finding an alternative mode is the answer. We need to look closely at the driven-doing mode of mind and see if we can spot any regular features that tell us discrepancy-based processing is operating and, if so, whether it is giving rise to problems. *We need to detect the tell-tale signs of the doing mode in general and the driven-doing mode in particular.* It turns out that there are commonly *seven* ways the doing mode reveals itself (see *The Mindful Way Workbook*, by Teasdale, Williams, & Segal, 2014, for further description). We summarize them in the sidebar on page 57 and point out how doing mode can easily become driven-doing.

The seven aspects of driven-doing work in concert to try to make things different from how they are. Changing things becomes

THE SEVEN SIGNS OF DOING MODE
AND HOW EACH CAN BECOME DRIVEN-DOING

1. **Automatic pilot:** Doing mode often comes on line automatically, so we do not see it operating. Driven-doing uses ordinary "doing" and problem solving as a stepping-stone to driven-doing. For example, a project you are working on might, at first, simply be a "project with milestones." However, when a deadline is approaching, notice how easily (and without conscious awareness) you become driven by it—it can come to seem *absolutely critical* and dominate your whole life for days at a time. In this state, you may commonly find that you do not taste your food, hear the birds, or see smiling children.

2. **Living in the head:** Doing mode uses thoughts and ideas to try to solve the problems it is working on. In driven-doing, these thoughts seem more urgent: there is a sense that more is at stake—our worth and integrity as a person seems now to depend on figuring out why things are why they are and why they can't be different.

3. **Mental time travel:** Doing brings back the past and imagines possible futures to help get where we want to be. In driven-doing, the mind is obsessive about reliving the past or preliving the future, and negative aspects of future and past color the whole mood of the present.

4. **Avoidant:** Doing mode keeps in mind what to avoid—where we *don't* want to end up. In driven-doing, the states a person wants to avoid are more negative, global, and self-referent (e.g., "I desperately don't want to feel so helpless ever again. If I do, I'll not be able to stand it. It'll show me for certain that things will never get better").

5. **Needs things to be different**. Doing mode works on strategies to resolve mismatches, forever monitoring the gap between where we are and where we want to be. In driven-doing, such monitoring is more persistent and "adhesive" because it seems to involve issues that are fundamental for the self.

6. **Thoughts as real:** Doing mode assumes that thoughts/ideas always tell the truth, since in most ordinary situations this is the case. The more toxic thoughts of driven-doing are also assumed to be true, even if they are thoughts such as, "No one wants me around anymore; I'm just a burden to my family and friends." "Killing myself is the only solution."

7. **Depletion:** Left to itself, doing continues to focus on the goal until it is reached, or until we are too tired to continue. Driven-doing ignores the cues that tell us we are too tired, since completing the goal is seen as much too important to let go of.

the major, preoccupying task. The person cannot let it go, the mind returns again and again to the same theme. It feels the most important thing in the world, and although sufferers may seem cheerful with family and friends, they feel as if they are playacting—underneath the mask they cannot wait to be by themselves to continue the rumination.

> It is not the doing mode that is the problem, but rather when the goals it is seeking (or the outcomes it is avoiding) become so engrossing and important to the sense of the worth and integrity of the self that the person desperately *needs* something to be a certain way—*driven-doing*.

Notice that driven-doing is one variant of the ordinary doing mode that all of us use everyday to get tasks done, so you can use this mode coming on line as a major opportunity. Week by week in an MBCT program, the teacher encourages participants to look out for the signs of doing mode in *ordinary* everyday life, then invites people to see if the mode is beginning to tip into driven-doing, and if so, to practice "nipping it in the bud" by switching to an alternative way of relating to themselves and the world. This alternative mode of mind has been called the mode of "being": intentional, experiential, present-moment-focused, seeing aversion clearly, allowing things to be as they are, seeing thoughts as mental events, and befriending the body/mind, ensuring it gets the nourishment it needs to flourish.

Being mode (see the sidebar on p. 59) does not bring all activity to a standstill. Rather, it entails waking up to what is happening as it is happening; seeing if it is possible, without critical self-judgment, to notice if what you are doing is what you had *intended* to be doing or whether functional doing has become "driven-doing." It involves seeing clearly that you can choose to switch from living in your head to a more embodied stance, if only for a moment, before reentering the world of busyness.

In each aspect of the driven-doing and alternative "being" mode, the practice of shifting from doing to being involves prioritizing bodily sensations. Here we give example items. After each item in this list, we indicate the session or class of the MBCT program that includes exercises focused on that item, for example:

- The touch, sight, smell, and taste of a raisin (Session 1).
- The raw physical sensations of the body lying down (Sessions 1 and 2).
- The physical sensations of the body as it moves (Session 3).
- The sensations of breathing and the body as a whole as it sits (Session 3 onward).
- The sensations that come along with pleasant and unpleasant moments during daily life (home practice after Sessions 2 and 3).
- Noticing sounds as a gateway to noticing thoughts and feelings as they arise and fade (Session 4).

THE BEING MODE OF MIND: AN ALTERNATIVE TO DRIVEN-DOING

1. From automatic pilot, participants learn to switch to becoming more **intentional**, conscious of what they are doing as they are doing it.

2. From living in their heads, people learn deliberately to shift to a **direct sense of the body.**

3. From reliving the past and preliving the future, people learn how to shift to **being fully in the present moment** (there is no need to switch off past and future, but now people *know* they are remembering, and *know* they are planning).

4. From trying to avoid, escape, or get rid of unpleasantness, people learn to switch to **approaching aversion with interest**: noticing what thinking, feeling, body sensations, and impulses are present.

5. From being hooked on to needing things to be different from how they are, people learn to **notice *where* in the body the problem is arising, and specific ways they can *allow things to be*** just as they find them.

6. From being entangled in thinking, taking thoughts personally, and seeing them as true, people learn how to shift to **seeing thoughts as *mental events*** that come and go moment by moment, often born out of unrecognized feelings.

7. From getting exhausted by preoccupation and chronic worry, people learn how to move deliberately from treating themselves harshly to **taking care of themselves with kindness**—even at times (*especially* at times) when they don't feel like doing so.

- Seeing what sensations in the body accompany any difficulty as it is deliberately held in mind (Session 5).
- The sensations in the body that reveal the feelings that give birth to (and disguise) negative thoughts (Session 6).
- The sensations that act as a warning sign that mood is deteriorating (Sessions 6 and 7).
- The sensations that warn that energy is getting depleted and signals the need to find specific ways of nourishing ourselves (Session 7).

The Science of Embodiment: Why Is the Body So Important?

"The damage done to us during our childhood cannot be undone, since we cannot change anything in our past. We can, however, change ourselves. we can . . . gain our lost integrity by choosing to look more closely at the knowledge that is stored inside our bodies and bringing this knowledge closer to our awareness" (Miller, 2007, p. 2).

Experiments on what happens when we pay sustained and friendly experiential attention to the raw sensations in the body, moment by moment, have led to extraordinary discoveries in both first-person accounts and third-person cognitive science experiments. In experiments pioneered by Watkins and Teasdale, different modes of mind are induced by instructing participants to imagine several states of mind, rather like the tiredness experiment you did earlier in the chapter (see pp. 51–53). In one experimental condition, participants think about "the *causes, meanings, and consequences*" of the state of mind they have been asked to imagine, thus encouraging a conceptual, analytic focus. In a second condition, participants "focus attention on the *experience*" of this state, thus encouraging a direct moment-to-moment focus.

Results show that these different modes of processing—analytic or experiential—dramatically affect the cognitive and emotional consequences of such focusing on the self. For example, experiential mode increases autobiographical memory specificity (Crane, Barnhofer,

Visser, Nightingale, & Williams, 2007), enhances problem-solving ability (Watkins & Moulds, 2005), speeds emotional recovery from a laboratory-induced negative event (Watkins, Moberly, & Moulds, 2008), and decreases estimation of weight gain in participants with an eating disorder (Rawal, Williams, & Park, 2011). This last example is particularly telling, since people with eating disorders are often said to be *over*focused on body, weight, and shape. But distinguishing an analytic focus on the body from an experiential focus on the body leads to a totally new hypothesis: that eating disorders such as anorexia involve overfocus on the *idea* of the body, but too little *experiential* processing of the raw sensations of the body itself. Our experiments have tested this hypothesis, showing that if experiential processing is induced, people suffering from anorexia no longer react catastrophically to the stress of imagining eating a large meal. Usually, even *imagining* such a meal makes sufferers believe they are heavier than they actually are. After practicing experiential processing for a few minutes, this reaction is not apparent or is much reduced (Rawal et al., 2011).

> The major aims of mindfulness training include, first, to learn to recognize the mode of mind that is currently operating (doing, driven-doing, or being); second, to see clearly whether it is the appropriate mode for the task in hand; and third, to give people the skills to switch out of the discrepancy mode of processing and enter an alternative mode of mind.

The alternative, experiential mode (the "being" mode of mind) uses the body for a number of reasons in both MBSR and MBCT:

- It facilitates remaining in the present moment. No one can focus *directly* on sensations in the body that happened in the past or will happen in the future; body sensations arise in the present.
- The body is an important source of information about the mind, so it can act as an early warning sign of impending mood shifts.
- It allows direct and unmediated perception: so perception does not need to be "refracted" through the lens of old schemas/ideas/attitudes/expectations.
- It helps people to see thoughts and mind states as mental events. When people learn to anchor the attention in the body, it gives a

"place to stand" from which they can see thoughts and feelings coming and going.

- It allows people to see the "feeling-tone" that accompanies each perception, action, and thought more clearly.
- It brings awareness and choice to the "leverage point" where feeling-tone turns into a strong impulse or urge to take immediate action, the precise point in the loop where an unattended bodily reaction would normally affect the mind's judgments and reactions in the next moment.

When we started this research, we wondered if we might come up against serious resistance to cultivating direct awareness of the body. Resistance can happen in any class, and although we witnessed it in our classes of suicidal people, our impression was that it was not any more of an issue than for any other class. We shall return to the issue when we describe our classes session by session in Chapters 7–14. For now, consider that although the body will often have been the locus of trauma for any who have experienced sexual or physical abuse, the practices in any mindfulness course invite participants to go at their own pace, to be very gentle with themselves, and to contact the teacher at any time if there are specific issues that they would like to discuss. If there are difficulties in moving attention to some sensitive regions of the body, then it is always possible to continue the practice using those parts of the body that are felt to be "safer" or "neutral" (e.g., for some, the soles of the feet; for others, the tip of the nose), so people need not feel excluded.

The Cultivation and Application of Being Mode

It is beyond the scope of this book to review the many ways in which mindfulness-based interventions help people suffering from a wide range of distressing physical and mental health conditions. The classic format developed by Kabat-Zinn involves eight weekly classes and home practice between sessions. In some mindfulness-based interventions a different pattern of classes is used: longer or shorter classes, fewer or more than eight classes, with follow-up classes or not. Whatever the exact course format, participants always receive extended training in (1) attentional focus and (2) open acceptance of whatever external and internal stimuli might arise, whether unpleasant or pleasant, from moment to moment (3) using open-hearted attending to the sensations arising in the body as foundational, anchoring people again and again in the present moment.

Mindfulness meditation helps people to distinguish primary sensory and cognitive experiences (body sensations, thoughts, images, feelings) from secondary emotional or cognitive reactivity to this experience. By learning to "allow" unpleasant experience and by cultivating stability in attention, participants learn meta-awareness, a direct "knowing" of when the mind is wandering (being "captured" by thoughts, feelings, and impulses), together with the ability to disengage from such modes of mind when they become ruminative, and to bring attention back to the intended focus. In this way, the mental training undermines the habitual tendency to bring on line the maladaptive driven-doing mode that tends to withdraw into brooding or worrying in reaction to negative physical or psychological events.

As described in *Mindfulness-Based Cognitive Therapy for Depression* (Segal et al., 2002, 2013), MBCT was specifically designed to help people who were at increased risk of relapsing back into serious clinical depression by targeting the mode of processing that people use when their mood begins to deteriorate. Entering the experiential "being" mode of processing at such times allows people to disengage from the relatively "automatic" ruminative thought patterns that attempt to fix things, and allows them to relate differently, more compassionately, to previously avoided negative material (see Segal et al., 2013; Teasdale, Williams, & Segal, 2014).

Many randomized controlled trials—carried out all over the world— have evaluated MBCT in depression. We shall return to these in the final chapter, for when we started the 10-year program of work described in this book (in 2003), there was only a single trial of MBCT (Teasdale et al., 2000). Yet the 2000 trial was critically important: It showed that MBCT could reduce the recurrence rate of the most recurrent patients over 12 months by 40–50% compared with usual care. Relatively soon after we started our work, a second study by Ma and Teasdale replicated this result (Ma & Teasdale, 2004), and the United Kingdom's National Institute for Clinical Excellence recommended MBCT as a cost-effective treatment for preventing relapse in depression. Other trials since that time have found that MBCT also helps people suffering from other problems: serious health anxiety, agoraphobia and chronic depression that is not responding to other treatments, persistent conditions such as tinnitus or chronic fatigue syndrome, and is showing promising results in helping to improve quality of life in those suffering from serious physical illness such as cancer as well as the most serious mental health difficulties such as bipolar disorder (see "Extending the Reach of MBCT Beyond Depressive Relapse" in Chapter 19 of Segal et al., 2013). However, it was the extension of MBCT to suicidal depression that was our central concern.

"So, How Can MBCT Help Me?"

The question is most likely to be asked first in the preclass interview when people decide whether to embark on a course. Chapter 6 goes into this in more detail, but our discussion of modes of mind clearly suggests a framework for how teachers may respond wisely to such a question.

First, recall that when difficult thoughts or memories come to mind, one of the reasons people get stuck is because the mind is using a strategy that is entangling things rather than helping. If this is true, you would expect this strategy to lead to despair and helplessness, for the mind has never been taught another way. And this will be especially true in people who are prone to depression who are likely to make the assumption that nothing can help and therefore nothing can change for the better.

MBCT teaches us to recognize when this is happening, and a *new* way of responding. But notice that the mind is doing the best it can. Participants do not need to add an extra layer of feeling bad on top of their existing feelings; participants feel helpless and trapped because the mind works in the way that it does.

> People get entangled when the mind uses a strategy that is inadvertently making things worse. This leads to despair and helplessness. Compassion arises when we realize that the mind does not know any different—it has never been taught another way.

Second, participants may recognize the way in which little things can trigger a cascade of emotion. MBCT trains people to see this more clearly, and earlier in the sequence. Third, if someone wants to know if there is evidence that this works, it is perfectly okay to say that research all over the world converges on the conclusion that MBCT reduces the risk of recurrence of depression, so it reduces one of the major factors that can lead to a sense of there being no hope. It also reduces anxiety, one of the major factors that can lead to strong urges to act on suicidal thoughts. It can help increase problem-solving skills because people find they can stand back a little from their difficulties and see things from other perspectives, and it helps people get better and more restful sleep. Chapter 18 will add particularly telling evidence to this picture.

If these issues arise in the preclass interview, however, we also balance enthusiasm with caution. We say that much depends on commitment to attend classes and carry out practice at home, and that this can seem difficult at times. Following our pilot research for people at risk of suicide, we added to this discussion in important ways (see Chapter 6), and we describe data showing how important practice turns out to be in Chapter 18.

Although in our early work with MBCT we were careful not to be too optimistic, or to give false hope to people about what outcome they might expect for themselves (we were concerned that participants would look for early signs of progress then get disappointed), we gradually came to realize we were in danger of being too cautious. Telling people not to raise their expectations didn't work anyway, and although we still say that the effects may take time to emerge, it is fine to say that virtually everyone who comes to class has found some benefit, and for many it has been transformative, making a huge difference to their lives. Encouraging hope is a central aspect of the first encounter with patients suffering from depression, and all the more so when suicidal despair is part of the picture.

> There is no need to dampen expectations. Virtually everyone who comes to class has found some benefit, and for many it has been transformative.

Concluding Remarks

The same questions, "So will this work for me? Can this work for me?", can come up in later sessions. The downside to being optimistic at the outset is that such early optimism can seem to increase the sense of frustration, struggle, doubt, and "here we go again" sense of hopelessness. Giving too ready an answer to such questions, asked at a point when things seem not to be "working as hoped," is not appropriate if this means that we thereby ignore the chance to explore the participant's hopelessness and doubt. It may be putting it too strongly to say this is what a teacher hopes for, but it remains true that it is important that when doubt, anger, struggle, and hopelessness happen in class, the experienced teacher recognizes that this despair is disclosing the central problem, and meeting such despair openly, with gentleness and curiosity, is what is called for. Despite the voice at the back of any teacher's mind saying anxiously "What is the most skillful thing to say here?", when profound hopelessness and turmoil come to the fore, there may be a deep knowing that, yes, this is it—this is the work we are here to do. The rest of this book aims to give the foundations for working with just such mental pain within MBCT.

PART II

MBCT FOR THOSE AT RISK OF SUICIDE

CHAPTER 5

Assessing Vulnerability
to Depression and Suicidality

MBCT teachers, like teachers of other mindfulness-based interventions, as far as possible, want to meet participants in an open atmosphere unbiased by expectations or preconceived notions. Nonetheless, it is helpful in understanding participants' inner worlds and in navigating the mindfulness training itself (in particular perhaps the inquiry process) to know about participants' psychological vulnerabilities. The main aim of this chapter is to provide an overview of the signs and signatures of the psychological processes involved in vulnerability and to describe ways in which teachers can gather information about them. The main focus in this context naturally is on vulnerability for relapse to depression and suicidal ideation. Furthermore, seeing that in patients who have suffered from suicidality in the past suicidal crises may easily escalate, it is also important for teachers to be able to discern risk for suicidal ideation to transfer into suicidal behavior. While a detailed discussion of risk assessment for suicidal behavior is beyond the scope of this chapter (see Hawton, Casañas, Comabella, Haw, & Saunders, 2013, for an overview of risk factors), we provide an outline of relevant factors and describe the practical procedures that we have put into place in our own work to respond to suicidality and to assure the safety of our participants.

When it comes to working with people who are highly vulnerable, the ability to recognize potential warning signs of impending crisis is essential for ethical practice. Teachers need to be familiar with such signs and have a good understanding of how to respond to them. This is why good practice guidelines demand that teachers who work specifically with highly vulnerable groups need appropriate clinical training and experience. And, given the high prevalence of depression and suicidality, even those who are offering classes that are not specifically for vulnerable patients may benefit from familiarizing themselves with potential warning signs and their assessment, as they may need to advise participants to seek professional help. We look at assessment in an inclusive sense here. "Assessment" involves "taking account" in either formal or informal ways, of the risks and vulnerabilities of participants, as well as the assets and strengths that have seen them through crises in the past. Importantly, assessment is not just a "one-time" process at the outset of a mindfulness-based intervention, but also an active discernment by the teacher, week by week, of the issues that are arising for participants as they learn to relate differently to the patterns of mind that have been so destructive in the past.

> Assessment is an active discernment by the teacher, week by week, of the issues that are arising for participants as they learn to relate differently to self-destructive patterns of mind.

In engaging in this process, it is helpful to have in mind a conceptual framework of the psychological processes that feed vulnerability, and of how the skills taught in mindfulness classes can most beneficially address these. Just as importantly, teachers need to be able to relate this theoretical knowledge to actual presentations in the classroom situation. A purely intellectual grasp of factors involved is of no value, unless it is accompanied by a deep sense of how they are experienced and felt by participants, and how to respond sensitively and wisely when they show themselves. This "gut-level" understanding comes most powerfully from being mindfully present with participants, not from reading books and articles on vulnerability. What exactly do I need to look out for as a teacher, in order to understand vulnerabilities in particular participants? What is the nature and feel of these when they become apparent in participants' behavior and in what they say about their experience in and outside of the classroom? As teachers, we learn about these aspects through mindful observation and relating. Yet, an understanding of conceptual backgrounds can help teachers' observations and crucially inform the process of developing a sense of what clues to look out for when observing and listening to participants in interviews and classes, to develop eyes and ears for tell-tale signs. Above all, teachers need to remain open to what is being brought into the class at any given moment. However, a firm conceptual foundation might help to facilitate openness for what might be hiding under the surface without predicting or suggesting it: be prepared to provide room for it to be seen, known, and met. This is particularly important when working with patients suffering from suicidal feelings, where shame and avoidance are common, and where allowing space for what is difficult to say in classes is especially relevant. Familiarity with the psychological instruments used to measure vulnerability can offer a starting point for cultivating a deeper understanding of these processes and how they play out in the experience of participants.

In clinical trials, recognizing vulnerabilities and strengths is helped by formal assessments of diagnostic status and history, through the use of standardized instruments such as structured clinical interviews and self-report questionnaires. These instruments have been developed to provide valid reflections of the psychological factors involved in vulnerability to depression and suicidality and are potentially illuminating not just for researchers and teachers, but also for participants themselves. Reflecting on their own responses to questions posed at a preclass or assessment interview offers an opportunity for participants to begin to decenter, to recognize characteristic old patterns, and see clearly that, if someone has been able to validate these instruments in many different people in many different clinics across the globe, these patterns which feel so utterly personal and true must in fact be shared by other people.

However, we are aware that using these instruments requires time and resources, which in many clinical settings are limited. Compared to clinical trials, classes provided in the contexts of day-to-day clinical practice may leave little time and room for formal assessment. Nonetheless, it seems recommendable and is certainly part of our own practice, to use at least brief measures of symptoms and core cognitive vulnerabilities on a weekly basis during the training in order to monitor changes, particularly when working with larger groups of patients where opportunities to hear about an individual's current state during classes are more restricted. For this purpose, we usually invite participants to come to the classes earlier, and to spend some time before the actual beginning of the class reflecting on the events of the past week by going through a brief set of questionnaires.

Let us move on now to see what measures can be used for this purpose. We will begin our overview of the signs and signatures of vulnerabilities and the ways in which these can be assessed by looking more closely at the marker of vulnerability that has been used to define the indication for MBCT. This will provide us with a more detailed understanding of the historical factors that may be involved in the development of vulnerability for recurrent depression.

Who Is Most Vulnerable?

The first two trials on MBCT (Ma & Teasdale 2004; Teasdale et al., 2000) confirmed what previous studies had found: the most consistent predictor of risk of relapse was the number of previous episodes of depression. But Teasdale et al. (2000) and Ma and Teasdale (2004) found a number of *other* important characteristics of those with more prior episodes, each of which provide a teacher with further indicators of vulnerability. First, those patients who experienced a greater number of prior episodes had an *earlier age of first onset* of major depression, so that their total length of history of depression was considerably longer than those with only two prior episodes (20 years vs. 5 years). Second, Ma and Teasdale (2004) showed that for those patients who had experienced more prior episodes any recurrence of depressive symptoms was more likely to come out of the blue—to be *autonomous*. Third, those with more episodes had significantly more trauma and adversity before the age of 16. Their parents were more *indifferent* (perceived as "uncaring of me," "rejecting of me," "ignoring me"), *abusive* ("verbally abusive of me," "unpredictable toward me," "physically violent or abusive of me"), or *overcontrolling* ("overprotective," "overcontrolling of me," "sought to make me feel guilty"; Parker et al., 1997). Segal et al. (2010) added an additional predictor of vulnerability that it is useful for teachers to know of. In their study, they found that those with an *unstable* pattern of remission (i.e., one week the symptoms would seem to have disappeared, only for them to reappear the next) had a higher risk of recurrence over the next 18 months.

This pattern of results from different studies suggests that those who are most vulnerable are those who are most reactive to small changes in mood. When there is a *long history of depression* that *starts early in life* and which in some people may even have involved *adversity and abuse as children*, then current mood shifts bring back toxic patterns from the past that seem to be relevant now, and create *unstable mood*. It is really helpful to keep this in mind when discerning what issues are present for someone at a preclass interview. The 8-week course has only a limited window of time to begin to taste how mindfulness might address these problems, so there is a strong need to make sure that the skills taught through the program address the processes most central to the persistence of the disorder.

Assessing Historical Markers of Risk

Characteristics of the course of the disorder can thus provide important initial pointers toward the vulnerabilities that patients harbor. In clinical trials, such information is usually assessed with structured clinical interviews, which are used to gather information relating to both past and present diagnoses, and thus also provide a picture of how current difficulties have developed over time. The most widely used of these interviews is the Structured Clinical Interview for DSM (SCID; First, Spitzer, Gibbon, & Williams, 2002). However, use of this standard research instrument requires considerable time, and may therefore not easily be feasible in many clinical contexts. This means that it may be necessary to rely on information gathered in a less formal way.

Visual Time Lines

In our diagnostic interviews for trials, we often use a visual time line to get an impression of the lifetime course of depression and suicidality. The time line consists of a simple horizontal line with age in years marked along it (see the box below). At right angles to it, there is a scale measuring mood (ranging from very bad to very good). We ask participants first to mark some anchor points (significant landmarks such as times when they lived in particular places or held particular jobs). Then we ask them to indicate episodes of depression by rating their mood at the time at which they felt worst during a given episode and marking that point. Finally participants join up these points by tracking their mood along the line, and additionally they indicate points at which they felt suicidal. The end result is a line providing a broad picture of the course of the depression and suicidality over the person's lifetime.

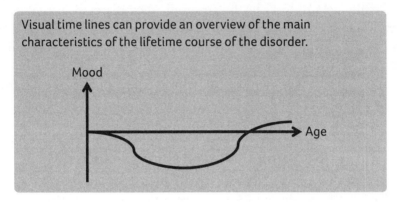

Visual time lines can provide an overview of the main characteristics of the lifetime course of the disorder.

By providing information about the onset of the depression, the number of lifetime episodes, and whether patients tend to be completely well between episodes or whether their symptoms tend to be more chronic, time lines offer a useful and easily accessible overview of the most relevant aspects of a person's course of depression and suicidality throughout the lifespan. In fact, recent research has shown that such broad-brush categorizations of lifetime course are much better at discriminating patients with high and low vulnerability than categorizations based on definitions from current diagnostic systems (Mondimore et al., 2007).

Because time lines are completed in dialogue with the participant, they allow teachers to get a sense of the circumstances under which episodes developed, and in the case of early episodes may therefore also provide information about childhood adversity. Self-report questionnaires can be used to supplement an interview in the assessment of early experiences. They can feel less intrusive than an interview and have been proven to be equally reliable in this context (Bernstein et al., 2003). A well-established instrument in this domain is the Child-hood Trauma Questionnaire (CTQ; Bernstein & Fink, 1998), which assesses the degree to which participants have been exposed to traumatic conditions during their early years. The questionnaire screens for traumatic events and background conditions that might surround such events. It asks about emotional, physical, and sexual abuse (such as feeling hated, being a target for hurtful remarks in the family, being badly hit, being punished with hard objects, being touched sexually or made to do sexual things), as well as signs of physical and emotional neglect (e.g., not feeling loved, not being looked out for, not being taken care of, or not having enough to eat), and therefore provides information not only about traumatic events but also about stressful background conditions. Example items include "I had to wear dirty clothes" (physical neglect), "I got hit or beaten so badly that it was noticed by someone like a teacher, neighbor or doctor" (physical abuse), "My family was a source of strength and support" (emotional neglect, reverse scored), "People in my family called me things like 'stupid,' 'lazy,' or 'ugly'" (emotional abuse), and "Someone tried to touch me in a sexual way or made me touch them" (sexual abuse). When giving this questionnaire to participants it is of course important to allow time to follow it up with dialogue.

Even where it is not possible for thorough formal assessments to be carried out, familiarity with the domains and items of this questionnaire might guide ideas about what to look out and listen for, particularly when it comes to building an impression of the background conditions that might have established chronic sources of stress of the kind that can have lasting and pervasive effects on how people relate to themselves and others (see the sidebar below).

Information about the course of depression and experiences surrounding the occurrence of early episodes might thus help to provide a more complete picture of what has prompted participants to come to

---

THE IMPACT OF EARLY TRAUMA

Research has clearly shown that early trauma and abuse can be associated with significant deficits in physical functioning in adulthood, including deficits in immunological functioning and increased endocrinological stress responses (Danese & McEwen, 2012). There is also evidence that early trauma is associated with alterations in brain structures critical in the processing of bodily sensations (Heim et al., 2013), possibly occurring as a consequence of tendencies to avoid bodily sensations or avoiding bringing awareness to particular regions of the body.

the classes. However, all of these factors—early adversity and trauma, early onset, a high number of previous episodes, chronic course—are historic in nature. So it is not possible to change them, nor are they in themselves the actual vulnerabilities. They are merely *pointers toward psychological vulnerability*, important only insofar as they provide insights into the actual expressions of vulnerability. The actual vulnerability is to be found in the psychological scars left behind, such as recurrent *themes* in thinking (e.g., finding it hard to trust others); particular *qualities* in how thoughts and feelings present themselves (e.g., feelings of anger or shame, and a strong tendency to avoid and suppress); particular *conclusions* (e.g., a sense that such thoughts and feelings could *never* be worked with). After all, some thought patterns are so habitual and overrehearsed, some thoughts (such as "I am a burden to others") may be so familiar that they are not seen as thoughts—mental events—at all, but only as a reflection of how things really are, always have been, and always will be.

Teachers may find it helpful to know about these aspects of early experience, in order to help them respond to participants' reports of experiences, to notice and recognize small signs of larger themes, and to look out for difficulties in investigating them in meditation, difficulties that might manifest in a number of ways. Such vigilance for signs of early adversity is important since people may find it very difficult to talk about it. In fact, some of the effects of early trauma and stress may be difficult to access in words, and instead be predominantly reflected in aspects of bodily functioning.

Regardless of their knowledge of a participant's background, teachers need above all to be able to notice and recognize participants' current vulnerability, particularly in the case of vulnerability for suicidality. What are they?

Increasing Therapist/Teacher Awareness of Vulnerability for Suicide

Just as with vulnerability for depression in general, it is important to be aware that the full range of vulnerability for suicidality may become obvious only under conditions of negative mood and stress. Information about how a person responds under these conditions is very likely to be more relevant than what can be learned from their thinking and behavior in normal mood (see the sidebar below). As we have seen, in those who have been depressed before, reactivation of depressive thinking can occur in response to changes in mood so subtle that patients are often not aware at the time that a shift in processing has occurred, and only experience its consequences further down the line. In fact, engaging in maladaptive patterns of negative thinking without fully recognizing what is happening is one of the hallmarks of vulnerability.

The particular patterns of thinking that become reactivated are likely to differ depending on patients' learning histories. If patients have been suicidal in the past, suicidal thinking and related cognitive processes, such as hopelessness, despair, and deficits in problem-solving, are more likely to resurface in these patients when mood becomes low (Williams et al., 2005, 2008). It is helpful therefore to look at the particular profile of processes that become reactivated.

The Leiden Index of Depression Sensitivity (LEIDS; Van der Does & Williams, 2003) is a self-report instrument that is specifically

---

ASSESSING SUICIDALITY: SOME HELPFUL QUESTIONS

- Have you ever had any thoughts of just wishing that you were dead or wishing that you could go to sleep and never wake up?
- *Or:* Sometimes when people get to breaking point they feel like ending it all. Have you ever got to that point?
- *Or:* Sometimes people get so overwhelmed by things that they feel like killing themselves. Have you ever felt like that?
- In the past couple of weeks have you had even a single thought of killing yourself, even for a fleeting moment?
- How much of the time do you spend thinking about suicide—50% of the time, 80% of the time?
- What plans or preparations have you made for killing yourself?
- When you say "You lost it," exactly what do you mean? What did you do then?
- What would you do later tonight if you began to have suicidal thoughts again?
- What other ways have you thought about killing yourself?

Based on Shea (1999).

aimed at assessing these profiles. The questionnaire measures a number of different facets including the degree to which patients show hopelessness and suicidality (e.g., "When I feel down, I more often feel hopeless about everything"), acceptance and coping (e.g., "When in a sad mood, I am more creative than usual"), aggression or impulsivity (e.g., "In a sad mood, I do more things that I will later regret"), attempts to understand and control (e.g., "When I feel sad, I spend more time thinking about what my moods reveal about me as a person"), risk aversion (e.g., "When in a low mood, I take fewer risks"), and rumination (e.g., "When I feel sad, I spend more time thinking about the possible causes of my moods") when they are feeling sad. It thus provides a good sense of the broader spectrum of cognitive reactivity with some facets of reactivity (such as ruminative thinking or risk aversion) more common to many people and others (such as hopelessness and suicidal thoughts) more specific to people with particular learning histories.

Reactions to Suicidal Thinking

Whether or not suicidal thoughts, once activated, will spiral into crisis depends on how patients react to them. It is worthwhile therefore to also assess patients' general tendencies toward rumination about and avoidance of suicidal themes. Rumination and other maladaptive thinking patterns may arise as an automatic response to subtle changes in mood, but patients may consider that there are good reasons for engaging in them. For example, rumination may feel like an attempt at problem solving and can be difficult to distinguish from more adaptive, reflective thinking about difficulties. However, in the context of negative mood repetitive ruminations are likely to shade into an anxious or gloomy brooding on questions that imply self-criticism and blame. Thinking about "What am I doing to deserve this?" or "Why do I have problems other people don't have?" while in negative mood creates a sense of discrepancy between the current and desired states that will almost inevitably reinforce negative mood. Nolen-Hoeksema and colleagues' Ruminative Response Style Questionnaire (Treynor, Gonzalez, & Nolen-Hoeksema, 2003) distinguishes between adaptive reflection and maladaptive brooding. While items on the reflection scale, such as "Write down what I am thinking and analyze it" can sometimes indicate a more purposeful turning inward in order to facilitate problem solving, items on the brooding scale reflect the kind of "why" questions that can easily lead into self-criticism, such as "Why can't I handle things better?"

It is sometimes possible to see in MBCT sessions how ruminative processes can take hold in the entire class, for example, when individual participants talk about negative experiences in a way that leads into an expanding flow of memories or concerns, or when what one participant says triggers similar reports and memories in others. Sharing of experiences is often helpful, but the unfolding of ruminative processes in the classes is likely to have the same negative effects as elsewhere. This of course provides a valuable opportunity for the teacher to point out its presence and help participants to become aware of and "unpack" the process. A number of clues can help to reveal the presence of rumination. Certainly, repetitiveness is most noticeable and perhaps most helpful in identifying it. As participants often come to realize, going over an issue several times without making significant progress toward reaching a decision or taking an action is very likely a useful signal that ruminative brooding has taken hold and that disengaging from this kind of thinking would be a skillful maneuver. Ruminative thinking is usually general and abstract, a characteristic linked to the difficulties depressed patients have in retrieving specific autobiographical memories, which itself is related to deficits in social problem-solving ability, experiential avoidance, and deficits in cognitive control (Williams et al., 2007). In situations where formal assessment of rumination and overgeneral memory are not feasible, it can be useful therefore to notice how far participants' reports of their experiences drift into global descriptions of events, a sense of "always," "never," and "whenever I . . . ," rather than being reflections of specific observations tied to particular situations and experiences. Furthermore, rumination is avoidant in nature. While retaining a focus on a particular subject, its relation to this subject is to analyze and think about it (conceptual processing), rather than experiencing it directly (experiential processing). Perhaps this seems like a safer place from which to view things, yet paradoxically it reinforces the negative mood that prompted engagement with rumination in the first place.

It is helpful to notice how far participants' reports of their experiences drift into global descriptions of events, a sense of "always," "never," and "whenever I . . . ," rather than being tied to particular situations and experiences.

Avoidance

When toxic suicidal thoughts threaten to spiral out of control, it is natural that patients may attempt instead to suppress or avoid them. Unfortunately, although suppression may be successful in the short term, deliberately avoiding particular trains of thought requires constant vigilance ("Is it still here?"), which paradoxically keeps it in mind and is likely to increase rather than decrease its accessibility ("rebound" effects). Patients might thus experience a repeated resurfacing of negative thoughts, images, and accompanying feelings, despite—in fact, precisely *because of*—deliberate attempts to suppress them. Yet fear of being overwhelmed by distressing thoughts and images, or concerns that things may get worse and worse without attempts at control, can lead them to continue, redoubling their efforts despite rebounds, gradually exhausting their cognitive resources, and all the time unwittingly making the problem worse. These paradoxical effects are particularly likely when patients' cognitive resources have already been undermined by fatigue, exhaustion, or negative mood. The White Bear Suppression Inventory (WBSI; Wegner & Zanakos, 1994) is the most widely used instrument to measure such tendencies toward thought suppression, and includes items such as "There are things that I try not to think about" and "I often have thoughts that I try to avoid." In the context of working with highly vulnerable patients, it is worth exploring such questions (see Table 5.1) also more specifically with regard to suppression of suicidal thoughts and images (Hepburn et al., 2009).

Fear of being overwhelmed by distressing thoughts and images can lead people to redouble their efforts at suppression, gradually exhausting their cognitive resources, so unwittingly making the problem worse.

TABLE 5.1. The White Bear Suppression Inventory for Suicidal Ideation (WBSI-si)

When they feel really bad, some people find that they experience suicidal thoughts. The statements below describe some ways that people have reacted to their own suicidal thoughts, but everybody is different. When thoughts about suicide come into your mind, how do you feel about them? Please read each statement carefully, circling a number to indicate how much you agree with it (1 = strongly disagree, 2 = disagree, 3 = neutral, 4 = agree, 5 = strongly agree).

When I feel very low and things get too much for me:

1. My thoughts return frequently to the idea of suicide (Intrusion).
2. I cannot erase images of suicide that come to my mind (Intrusion).
4. Suicidal thoughts keep jumping into my head (Intrusion).
5. I wonder why I have the suicidal thoughts I do (Intrusion).
6. I wish I could stop thinking of suicide (Intrusion).
8. I try not to tell anyone about the suicidal thoughts I have (Intrusion).
9. I prefer not to think about suicide (Suppression).
10. I try to avoid suicidal thoughts (Suppression).
12. The suicidal thoughts sometimes come so fast I wish I could stop them (Intrusion).
13. I sometimes stay really busy just to keep suicidal thoughts from intruding on my mind (Distraction).
14. I have suicidal thoughts that I cannot stop (Intrusion).
16. I try not to think about suicide (Suppression).
17. I often do things to distract myself from my suicidal thoughts (Distraction)
18. My suicidal thoughts sometimes make me really wish I could stop thinking altogether (Distraction).
20. I always try to put suicidal thoughts out of mind (Suppression).

Note. The original adaptation of the WBSI scale also included five Comfort Items (i.e., items 3, 7, 11, 15, and 19) to be calculated as a separate measure, The Comfort Scale. From Williams, Duggan, Crane, and Hepburn (2011). Copyright 2011 by John Wiley & Sons, Ltd. Reprinted by permission.

The WBSI is mainly focused on suppression of thoughts. While this is an important domain, it is not only negative thoughts but also aversive feelings and body states that people tend to avoid. "Experiential avoidance" refers to the broader tendency to avoid internal experiences including thoughts, feelings, and bodily sensations, and can be assessed using the Action and Avoidance Questionnaire (AAQ; Hayes et al., 2004), which includes items to assess avoidance of feelings such as "I'm not afraid of my feelings," but covers an entire range of other aspects that might be associated with experiential avoidance in its stricter sense including avoidant behaviors, and cognitive responses such as worry and beliefs about emotions.

In the classroom, avoidance finds its expression in a number of different ways. In inquiries we often guide participants to explore the bodily sensations and feeling states that come with particular thoughts or memories, encouraging openness and curiosity about even difficult experiences. This practice, like all the meditation practices, tends to dissolve experiential avoidance, but it is not easy or straightforward (see Chapters 11 and 15), and it is often possible to observe, during such dialogues, hesitations or concerns relating to opening to experience that are indicative of experiential avoidance.

Assessing Suicidal Thinking

For those at risk of suicide, depression is potentially a fatal condition, and it is therefore a prime concern for teachers to assure participants' safety and well-being. MBCT classes offer few opportunities for individual contact between teacher and participants, so teachers need to think about other means of monitoring depression and suicidality in those who are highly vulnerable. As described in the introduction to this chapter, one way of doing this is regularly to gather indications of relevant warning signs through the use of brief questionnaires. Using weekly measures is now routine in many U.K. mental health settings, and in our trials we have asked participants before each session to fill in a set of scales that give an impression of their current symptoms and how much they engaged in rumination and suppression, as well as the degree to which they experienced intrusive imagery during the past week. Asking patients to fill in standard questionnaires for symptoms of depression such as the Beck Depression Inventory (BDI; Beck, Steer, & Brown, 1996) on a weekly basis and looking out for changes in items that assess hopelessness and suicidality is also good practice when working with groups of highly vulnerable patients.

Furthermore, it is helpful to think about ways of addressing suicidal thinking within the intervention. As participants go through the course, engaging in the meditation practices and cultivating increased mindfulness in their daily activities, they repeatedly encounter situations in which depressive thinking is activated, and in which they find their minds drawn into rumination, or engage in attempts to avoid and suppress negative memories and thoughts. These mental events stand out clearly during the steady attentional gaze of meditation, and thus offer repeated chances to practice recognizing and responding differently to unintended trains of thought. Thus what might otherwise be no more than distractions provide valuable opportunities for learning, for becoming familiar with the signs of vulnerability, and thus building a foundation for new ways of relating to negative mood and thinking. We sometimes refer to the wandering of the mind during meditation as "grist to the mill," and our experience from the classes is that, as teachers, we can trust that wandering into depressive thinking will occur frequently enough for this essential learning to occur.

This may not be true to the same degree for suicidal thinking. We have found in our research that, in those who have been suicidal in the past, suicidal thinking can be reactivated in very much the same ways as other forms of negative thinking (Williams et al., 2008). Yet participants seldom report it occurring spontaneously during meditations or in their daily life. Of course, as we have seen, this might in part be due to reluctance to report such thoughts, and in part it might be due to the fact that suicidal thinking may arise in images rather than verbal thoughts, and therefore be wrongly perceived as not within the realm of mental events that we refer to when we practice finding a different relation to negative thinking. Whatever the reason, however, the result is that what is most difficult to deal with has least opportunity to be practiced with. If suicidal thinking differs in some ways from other depressive thinking, this may be an important factor in knowing how best to respond to it. One way in which we have responded to this complication is by making changes to the program so that there is room to look not only at the territory of depression, but specifically at the territory of suicidality itself (see Chapter 11). At the same time, this observation is a reminder that it is important and listen out and watch for signs of suicidal thinking, and to be prepared to help participants to acknowledge and explore it through inquiry where this seems appropriate and helpful.

So teachers need to become familiar with the territory of suicidality, just as they are familiar with the territory of depression, both in terms of imagery and the verbal thinking that may come with it. A questionnaire that provides a good description of the verbal beliefs that drive suicidality is the Suicidal Cognitions Scale (SCS; Rudd, Joiner, & Rajab, 2001, see Table 5.2). These include *perceived burdensomeness* (e.g., "I am a burden to my family"), *helplessness* (e.g., "No one can help solve my problems"), *unlovability* (e.g., "I am completely unworthy of love"), and *poor distress tolerance* (e.g., "When I get this upset, it is unbearable"). Keeping in mind that such thinking can be easily reactivated in people with a history of suicidal depression, we have sometimes used the questions from this measure to ask patients how much they endorse these particular forms of thinking when they are in a negative mood, and also how much they are able to decenter from them, that is, to see them as thoughts and not as facts, when they occur.

The Orbach–Mikulincer Mental Pain Scale (Orbach, Mikulincer, Gilboa-Schechtman, & Sirota, 2003) is another questionnaire that describes judgments that, in a state of distress, may lead into a suicidal crisis, and thus provides reminders of warning signs to keep in mind when listening to participants experiencing distress. Orbach and colleagues differentiate the following facets of mental pain: sense of irreversibility ("I have lost something that I will never find again"), loss of control ("I have no control over the situation"), narcissist wounds ("I feel abandoned and lonely"), emotional flooding ("My feelings change all the time"), freezing ("I feel numb and not alive"), self-estrangement ("I feel that I am not my old self anymore"), confusion ("I have difficulties thinking"), social distancing ("I don't feel like talking to other people"), and emptiness ("I can't find meaning in my life").

As the research by our colleagues Emily Holmes and Catherine Crane suggests (Crane et al., 2012; Holmes et al., 2007), it may be particularly important in this context to look out for suicidal imagery. In their research, they used a structured interview in which they asked patients whether at a time at which they had been most despairing, they

TABLE 5.2. Suicidal Cognitions Scale

The following are 20 statements intended to assess your *current* problems. Please read each statement carefully and circle the number that best describes your thoughts right now. Remember to rate each item and circle only one number for each item (1 = strongly disagree, 2 = disagree, 3 = neutral, 4 = agree, 5 = strongly agree).

1. This world would be better off without me.
2. Suicide is my only option to solve my problems.
3. I can't stand this pain anymore.
4. I am a burden to my family.
5. I've never been successful at anything.
6. I can't tolerate being this upset any longer.
7. I can never be forgiven for the mistakes I have made.
8. No one can help solve my problems.
9. When I get this upset, it is unbearable.
10. I am completely unworthy of love.
11. Nothing can help solve my problems.
12. It is impossible to describe how badly I feel.
13. I have driven away everyone in my life.
14. I can't cope with my problems any longer.
15. I can't imagine anyone being able to withstand this unbearable pain.
16. There is nothing redeeming about me.
17. Suicide is the only way to end this unbearable pain.
18. I don't deserve to live another moment.
19. I would rather die now than feel this unbearable pain.
20. No one is as loathsome as me.

Note. From Rudd, Joiner, and Rajab (2001). Copyright 2001 by The Guilford Press. Reprinted by permission.

had experienced imagery (see the questions in Table 5.3). The suicidal imagery that was reported most often and that therefore seems most important to look out for is imagery "of yourself planning/preparing to harm yourself or make a future suicide attempt," "of what might happen to you if you died," "of what might happen to other people if you died," and "of things you were escaping from."

Strong endorsement of the above beliefs and presence of suicidal imagery indicates actual risk of suicide, and should act as a wake-up call to assess risk more thoroughly.

TABLE 5.3. Questions about Suicidal Imagery

When at your most despairing or suicidal, what images came to mind . . .

- Of a time you tried to harm yourself in the past?
- Of yourself planning/preparing to harm yourself or make a future suicide attempt?
- Of what might happen to you if you died?
- Of what might happen to other people if you died?
- Of things you were escaping from?
- Of another (nonsuicide related) distressing event that happened to you (e.g., a trauma)?
- That made you feel safe or better?
- That were fleeting/unclear?
- Any other type?

Can you tell me the *most significant image* you experienced when at your most despairing or suicidal?

Can you describe it in detail?

Does it have any other associations or meanings for you?

How *real* do these images feel (when at your most despairing) and how much *time* did you experience images specifically related to suicide (i.e., how preoccupying was it for you)?

Note. Pilot work indicated that suicide-related images may be comforting as well as distressing, so both can be explored. Questions from the structured interview used in the studies of Holmes, Crane, Fennell, and Williams (2007). Reprinted with permission from the authors.

Protective Factors

In the assessment of suicidality, risk factors (such as previous suicide attempts or ideation, current levels of depression, difficulties in impulse control, being single, and having a low level of education) have to be weighed against protective factors—in particular those factors that hold people back from suicidal behavior, even when they are highly distressed. Marsha Linehan and her colleagues have developed a questionnaire specifically to assess the importance of patients' reasons *not* to make a suicide attempt (Reasons for Living Inventory; Linehan, Goodstein, Nielsen, & Chiles, 1983). Domains of this questionnaire include survival and coping beliefs ("I still have many things left to do"), responsibility to family or friends ("It would hurt my family too much and I would not want them to suffer"), child-related concerns ("I want to watch my children as they grow"), fear of suicide ("I am afraid of the unknown"), fear of social disapproval ("Other people would think I am weak and selfish"), and moral objections to suicide ("My religious beliefs forbid it").

Presence of even just one of these reasons for living, be it that people fear the consequences for their loved ones or that suicide would violate their own beliefs, can be a powerful detriment to acting on suicidal ideation. It is really important for teachers and therapists to know what these positive reasons for living are, but also to get a sense of how fragile each of them is. As one participant said, "I would never actually kill myself while my dad is alive; but once he's gone, then there'll be no reason not to"

Responding to a Suicidal Crisis

What if there is significant cause for concern? What if participants report active or passive suicidal desire right now, that is, thoughts about actively hurting themselves or thoughts about being better off dead, or if they have actually made preparations to harm themselves. Any expression of suicidal feelings is traumatic for those who are feeling like this, and for those around them. For teachers, realizing that a

ASSESSING COGNITIVE VULNERABILITIES FOR DEPRESSION AND SUICIDALITY

Cognitive reactivity: The LEIDS (Van der Does & Williams, 2003) assesses reactivation of depressive and suicidal thinking; the Anxiety Sensitivity Inventory (ASI; Taylor et al., 2006) assesses responses to symptoms of anxiety.

Rumination, suppression, and avoidance: The RRSQ (Treynor, Gonzalez, & Nolen-Hoeksema, 2003) assesses maladaptive and adaptive forms of repetitive thinking; the WSBI (Wegner & Zanakos, 1994) assesses general tendencies to suppress negative thoughts; the AAQ (Hayes et al., 2004) measures general tendencies toward experiential avoidance.

Suicidal thinking and images: Suicidal thinking can be assessed using the SCS (Rudd et al., 2001) and the Orbach–Mikulincer Mental Pain Scale (Orbach et al., 2003); suicidal imagery may be explored in dialogue.

KEY STEPS IN PREVENTING AND RESPONDING TO SUICIDAL CRISIS

Monitoring: Tracking and monitoring participants' mood on a weekly basis during the course using brief questionnaires including items asking explicitly about current suicidal feelings.

Preparing: Making sure that participants have a crisis plan in place that is easy to follow through. Asking participants to fill in a crisis card in which they list three people they can contact in case of crisis.

Responding: Having agreed-upon procedures in place for teachers and staff to respond to suicidal feelings that specify how to assess current risk and how to proceed in order to make contact with relevant caregivers or emergency services.

patient is suicidal is an upsetting and fear-provoking experience, precisely because teachers care so much about their participants. It can be difficult in such situations to keep a clear head when such fear is around. It is helpful therefore for both participants and teachers to have thought about possible responses to suicidal feelings in advance, so that in case of crisis set procedures are in place to facilitate taking the necessary actions swiftly and with confidence. Having procedures in place to respond to suicidal crises (in a way that is congruent with the policy of the employing organization and the professional standards of the teacher) is part of good and ethical practice.

Developing a Crisis Plan

To this end, at the beginning of the process of engagement, either during the formal assessment process or during the preclass interview, we routinely invite participants to complete a crisis card. Here, they list up to three people whom they know they can contact in case of a crisis, and then make a concrete plan how they would go about doing this. The person they could contact could be a professional already involved in their care or someone close to them, a partner or family member or friend they felt they could trust. Participants fill in a card during the preclass session, and are invited to reflect further on their choices afterward, perhaps adding to or changing what they have written if they could see better options later. To make sure that in case of crisis participants can easily find their cards, we suggested they keep them right at the front of their course materials. We spend time too ensuring that participants understand and remember the reason for making the card, and go back to it during Session 2 of the MBCT course in order to review and refresh the memory of it. At this point we also invite them to add things that they could do to soothe themselves, and to list people whom they could contact under different circumstances. For example, there may be some friends they could contact simply because they know "this person is good for me" ("She makes me feel good and we don't talk about our problems"). There may be others they contact specifically because they *want* to be able to talk openly (and this might include previously listed professional helpers, as well as those friends, family, and others who know about their difficulties).

Preparing a crisis plan in this way is an important preemptive step. In the midst of a crisis, perfectly viable options might seem hopeless and people might find it hard to believe that anything would help. Having a specific, concrete plan that they had made when well helps participants to help themselves, even when they are feeling utterly trapped by their emotional pain and turmoil.

Developing a Risk Protocol for Staff

Similarly, for our own guidance, we have a protocol in place specifying how to respond when there is a reason to believe that participants are at risk of suicidal behavior or self-harm (see Table 5.4 for circumstances that should raise concern). The protocol describes how to proceed, from the initial assessment of risk to the involvement of other caregivers and emergency services if someone has already harmed him- or herself. It is put into action whenever there are concerns about suicidal feelings that seem overwhelming, that is, when people report a strong desire to kill themselves, have continuous thoughts about suicide, have a suicide plan, say they have recently made a suicide attempt, or are suffering from severe symptoms that significantly increase risk of suicidality (e.g., severe mania or psychosis) (see Table 5.4).

TABLE 5.4. Circumstances That Should Raise Concern and Questions to Gather Further Information

Concern should be raised in circumstances such as those in which participants report:
- A strong desire to kill themselves.
- Continuous thoughts about killing themselves.
- Having a suicide plan.
- Being sure they will make a suicide attempt.
- Has recently made a suicide/self-harm attempt.
- Severe manic or psychotic symptoms.

When suicidal feelings seem overwhelming, gather information about professional help the person is currently receiving. If the person is on the telephone, this involves inquiring, "Where are you now?" and under all circumstances to ascertain:
- "How long have you been having suicidal thoughts?"
- "Have you done anything to harm yourself?"
- "Have you shared your thoughts with anyone else?"
- "Have you talked to your family doctor or any other professional about this?"

The teacher needs to be aware that shame, self-hatred, emotional turmoil, and other reasons might initially lead participants in crisis to reject our offer to help and to involve others. So, if what participants tell us raises concern, we openly acknowledge this and tell them that, even though they might not feel comfortable about it, we have a professional and ethical obligation to take action to protect them. At the same time, it is crucial to remain in a respectful and understanding contact with them, assuring them that what is most important to us is their safety and well-being and that this is our only reason for overriding their wishes. In most situations, the priority is to persuade participants to contact their general practitioners (GPs), who in the United Kingdom act as the first port of call for medical interventions and who are responsible for initiating further action, including the involvement of crisis teams and, if necessary, hospitalization. It is preferable, of course, if participants make this contact themselves, and we would encourage them to do so. At the same time, the protocol specifies that we ask their permission either to follow up their call or to make initial contact with their GP ourselves. If this sensitive discussion between professional and participant is face to face, a good way of proceeding is to telephone the GP then and there, in the presence of the participant, so that they know exactly what is said. Where a participant does not give consent for the GP to be contacted, our procedures specify that we first discuss the case with a colleague, preferably involving a senior member of the team with extensive experience of working with depression and suicidality. If after that discussion the participant is still felt to be at serious risk, we would contact them again, express our concerns, and explain that we have no option other than to inform their GP even though they don't want us to. If in doubt, we always adopt a cautious approach and contact the GP. When we have spoken to family members after a loved one has committed suicide, one of the most difficult things for them to cope with is to discover that their loved one was known to be at serious risk by someone in the "professional" network, but that the risk was not communicated to anyone else so help was not provided.

Should a participant already have harmed him- or herself in some way, we respond depending on where they are and their current circumstances, call an ambulance, and then call the participant back and, if possible, continue talking to them until the ambulance arrives (see Table 5.5).

Naturally for other contexts, such standard procedures need adapting to the particular environment the work is conducted in, taking into account as many of the contextual factors as possible, including, for example, having all relevant contact information easily available. Even in contexts where risk might be considered relatively low, it is worthwhile having such procedures in place, as the occurrences they are designed to manage are difficult to predict.

Are There Contraindications?

Even though suicidal crises may be rare occurrences, providing classes for patients who are highly vulnerable means that participants and teachers will often be faced with the challenge of working with difficulties. Given their high levels of vulnerability, it is very likely that these participants will experience times when they feel sad, hopeless, or even suicidal again during the 8 weeks of the classes. And to a certain

TABLE 5.5. Teachers' Risk Protocol for When Participants Are at Risk of Suicide

The teacher should endeavor to ascertain information about the individual's current care plan (if there is one). For example, the teacher might ask:
- "When is your next appointment with your doctor?"
- "Could you contact your doctor today to talk about how you are feeling at the moment?"
- "Could you discuss this with your family members, friends?"

The teacher/assessor should openly indicate his or her concern about the person. The following areas can be communicated:
- "I am very concerned about your safety because you have expressed serious suicidal ideas."
- "While all the information you have provided as part of the course will remain completely confidential, it is my professional and ethical responsibility to take action to protect you if you are at serious risk of harm."

The teacher/assessor should strongly encourage the individual to make further contact with his or her GP:
- If the person agrees that the teacher may contact the GP, then this should be done in all circumstances. Action taken by the GP is at the GP's discretion.

If the person does not give permission for his or her GP to be contacted:
- The teacher should strongly encourage the individual to make contact him- or herself and discuss with other colleagues with clinical experience (named in the protocol) if they feel it might be necessary to go against the individual's wishes to contact his or her GP in the interests of safety.
- If it is felt that the person is at serious risk, then the teacher/assessor should express to the person that he or she is very concerned about his or her well-being, and that having discussed the situation with colleagues he or she feels he or she has no option but to contact the GP.

If an individual indicates that he or she has already harmed him- or herself:
- The teacher/assessor should try to ascertain the person's location and his or her circumstances, inform the person that his or her safety is a primary concern, call an ambulance, and inform other colleagues.
- The teacher should then call the person back and attempt to keep him or her talking until the ambulance arrives.

degree this might even be welcome as it provides participants with the opportunity to apply what has been learned in the classes to relevant events in their lives. Yet MBCT is a training of mental skills that comes with considerable demands. If participants are suffering from significant levels of symptoms, they might easily get overwhelmed rather than benefit from the practices. It is important therefore to discern how far participants will be able to follow the program. Teachers may respond to difficulties by helping participants to adjust the nature and amount of practice in order to keep patients engaged in the program even during difficult times. If difficulties with engaging in the practices occur and are an issue from the outset, this should be considered an important contraindication. Frequent reoccurrence of symptoms is a hallmark of vulnerability, and as research by Segal et al. (2010) has shown, participants with unstable remissions are particularly likely to show good response. Yet, if clinical levels of symptoms persist and continue to undermine patients functioning, other interventions are needed to support patients before they can engage in mindfulness training in a way that will bring beneficial effects.

Concluding Remarks

In this chapter we have provided an overview of the signs of vulnerability for depression and suicidality, the ways in which clinicians can prepare for swift responses to suicidal crises in order to facilitate identification, and responding to these characteristics.

People may differ in their inherent capacity for mindfulness and self-compassion, but stress and negative mood almost inevitably come with a decrease in mindfulness and, in the case of depression, a harshly self-critical pattern of thinking that can easily outweigh compassion toward the self. Yet it is exactly when people bring mindfulness and self-compassion to difficult situations that change becomes possible.

There is thus a particular dynamic between the psychological vulnerabilities we have described here and the resources that a mindfulness intervention provides. The rumination, suppression, and avoidance that keep negative mood in place often feed on a *lack* of mindfulness and self-compassion, while the healing qualities of mindfulness allow people to step back and disengage from these processes with kindness and compassion. The things that mindfulness seems particularly suited to address are thus the very same things that create the biggest barriers to engagement. As participants come to realize the detrimental effects of rumination and avoidance, so the beneficial effects of mindfulness and self-compassion become more obvious, just as it is in the most difficult of situations that we can see most easily how compassion "makes sense." As we will describe, conveying this understanding to our patients with suicidal depression was to be an important starting point, helping them engage with the program, even (or particularly) at times when they were feeling totally demoralized and trapped by the thought that things could never improve.

CHAPTER 6

Developing the Preclass Interview

*Encouraging Vulnerable Participants to Engage in
and Persist with Mindfulness Meditation*

Completing a course of MBCT, whether in a class or one-to-one with a therapist or teacher, necessitates an intense and sustained commitment from participants. They must set aside a substantial amount of time for home practice (up to 1 hour, 6 days out of seven, for at least 8 weeks). This in itself is often a challenge: How can it be fitted into a busy life and set alongside commitments to work and family? Perhaps more importantly for people who are particularly vulnerable, such as those who are recurrently suicidal, mindfulness meditation can seem to open a space in the mind into which anything can intrude—adverse events from the past, despair about the future. If what comes into the mind is painful and aversive, or if pain and aversion are barely held at bay by suppression or a flight into "fixing" mode and rumination, then this essential element of the program will present an even greater challenge. Engaging and continuing with this necessary work demands courage and persistence.

The central intention of the course is to learn to respond with steady kindness to difficult experiences, turning toward them and allowing them to be present, rather than trying to avoid them or analyze them out of existence. This change of stance is difficult enough for people with no particular emotional or psychiatric problems, dealing with everyday difficulties and upsets. How much harder it is for patients who are invited to make the same radical shift with the intense thoughts and emotions that fuel recurrent depression, let alone those whose depression has its roots in the pain of childhood adversity and abuse, and is accompanied by hopelessness, despair, and suicidal thoughts.

How can we encourage highly vulnerable participants to engage in and persist with the challenging work of mindfulness meditation training? This question came sharply into focus when we first offered MBCT for those who had been recurrently depressed alongside thoughts of killing themselves or even attempts at suicide. Let us look in more detail at what we had intended, what we did, and what we found that disturbed us.

Offering MBCT to Those at Risk of Suicide: First Steps

Over the early years of our research program, we first developed and piloted a version of MBCT we believed would be helpful for people who not only experienced recurrent depression, but who were also subject to despair and hopelessness, expressed by recurrent suicidal thoughts, feelings, or behaviors. Local GPs and our psychiatric colleagues referred to our clinic selected patients they knew to be at particular risk of suicide, and we offered MBCT to small classes of their patients, while they (GP or psychiatrist) retained clinical care and responsibility: an essential aspect of caring for people at such high risk. Mostly our program was closely based on the original classic MBCT course, but we rapidly found we needed to make some crucial changes to allow it to be more accessible to this particular group (details of the changes we made are given in Chapters 7–14). Once we had what seemed like a viable curriculum, we needed to establish whether it would indeed be helpful to the people we had in mind. So our second step was to conduct a relatively small-scale randomized controlled "pilot trial," in order to establish whether the program as it stood would be found feasible and acceptable by our participants. If not, we would need to think again.

The Pilot Trial

The pilot trial was carried out in Oxford. We recruited participants between the ages of 18 and 65 who had been well for at least 8 weeks, but who had in the past experienced at least one episode of major depressive disorder (MDD) and had a history of active suicidal ideation or had made a suicide attempt. We included people with a history of unipolar depression, as well as people with bipolar disorder, provided that the latter met the same criteria for depressive episodes as those with unipolar depression, and had not experienced a manic or hypomanic episode within the past 6 months. As cognitive-behavioral therapy (CBT) is known to have a relapse prevention effect (Hollon et al., 2005), we excluded people who had already undertaken a course of CBT unless their depression had since returned. We recruited 68 participants who matched the symptom pattern we were looking for and who were willing to be allocated on a random basis to receive an 8-week course of MBCT either immediately or after a delay. This would allow us to determine how helpful the revised program might be through a simple comparison of the two groups.

We conducted detailed clinical assessments when people entered the trial, including a structured diagnostic interview, the Structured Clinical Interview for DSM-IV (SCID; First et al., 2002), and a measure of depressed mood, the Beck Depression Inventory (BDI-II; Beck et al., 1996). In addition, we included a number of psychological assessments (questionnaires and laboratory tasks) which would allow us to assess the factors that we hypothesized were implicated in triggering the suicidal mode of mind in the presence of mild low mood and in promoting its escalation and persistence, and to evaluate the impact of the classes. All of these initial assessments were repeated for both groups after those allocated to receive immediate MBCT had completed the eight weekly classes.

Questionnaires

We used a questionnaire measure of rumination, the Ruminative Responses Subscale (RRS; Treynor et al., 2003), which assesses how people react when feeling low or depressed. Twelve items tap into rumination related to mood state (e.g., "Think about how hard it is to concentrate"), five assess "brooding" (e.g., "Why can't I handle things better?"), and five assess "reflection" which means pondering things in a way less likely necessarily to intensify distress (e.g., "Analyze recent events to try to understand why you are depressed"). Another questionnaire measure, a modified version of the Self-Description Questionnaire (SDQ; Carver, Lawrence, & Scheier, 1999), would evaluate how participants judged themselves *as they actually were* against their *ideal* selves, the selves they believed they *ought* to be, and the selves they *feared* they might be. This questionnaire taps into a pattern characteristically present in depression, known as "discrepancy-based processing": a relentless focus on shortcomings, and in particular on the gap or discrepancy between me as I am and me as I want or ought to be. Not surprisingly, this "mind the gap" thinking pattern feeds into low mood, as well as opening the door to fruitless ruminations about why I am the way I am, why I can't pull myself together, what is the matter with me, and so forth.

Laboratory Tasks

VULNERABILITY TO SUICIDALITY (COGNITIVE REACTIVITY)

One cognitive laboratory task was intended to measure cognitive reactivity, specifically how far participants' ability to identify potential solutions to interpersonal problems might be compromised in the presence of small amounts of low mood. To assess this, we used a modified version of the Means–End Problem-Solving Task (Platt, Spivak, & Bloom, 1978), which presents a number of problem situations (e.g., losing a watch, moving to a new neighborhood where you know no one), together with a happy ending to each story (you have found the watch, you have made new friends). The task is to think up as many ways as possible of bridging the gap between problem and happy ending. Participants' responses were then evaluated for their effectiveness by independent judges, and we assessed both how many responses were produced and how effective they were judged to be. Previous research had shown us that, while in recovery and in normal mood, previously suicidal patients were no different from other people in their problem-solving capacity, equivalent to people who had never been depressed and patients who had been depressed but *not* suicidal in the past. However, when we employed an experimental procedure that induced mild, transient low mood (listening to gloomy music while reading gloomy statements), problem-solving deficits emerged clearly. This was not true for the people who had been depressed in the past *without* suicidal thinking or behavior, even though the induction procedure had just as powerful an effect on their mood. Thus, we had discovered a vulnerability signature specific to suicidality, rather than true of depression in general. We now wanted to see if this process could be affected by MBCT. As it turned out, something happened that prevented us from finding out, as we'll discuss later.

NEUROLOGICAL FUNCTIONING (FRONTAL α-ASYMMETRY)

Second, with a smaller sample of MBCT ($n = 10$) and treatment-as-usual ($n = 12$) participants, we used a test of biological functioning—a measure of frontal α-asymmetry—that is considered to reflect approach and avoidance modes at a neurological level.

What We Discovered

Did MBCT Help?

Postclass comments suggested that participants had found the classes of value. Here is a selection of comments from participants who attended the eighth and final class:

- "Thank you for giving me my life back. I found my past was controlling my life, but now I know how to handle flashbacks and not let them interfere with my present. I'm looking at life through new eyes and enjoying it all over again. Now I am strong enough to really live my life" [participant with a history of childhood abuse who used the "sitting with the difficult" practice to begin to allow herself to recall and process her experiences].

- "This has been a very important course for me. It has taught me to try to find a space for myself, to value my own time. At first I felt guilty of being selfish, taking time from family and friends. Now I know that it's vitally important for me to do this. If I can't be there for myself, how can I possibly be there for others?"

• "This program has been extremely important to me. I came to it with very mixed feelings and considerable apprehensiveness. Now I feel much stronger and more capable than just 6 months ago. Such a sense of mutual support in the group—there is great value and strength to be drawn from shared human experience."

• "I have found the sessions both helpful and challenging— challenging my perceptions about my thoughts and where they take me, though I have struggled at times to acknowledge that they are only thoughts."

• "It's been useful in that, at times, I have managed just to 'be' rather than to be continually thinking and fretting."

• "I have been struggling for a very long time—years—with my 'self' and the world, life. Sorting out other people's problems and *not* my own. I finally found a time and place within myself to seek more help and support."

• "It has provided me with the means to make a choice—invaluable. I can observe a reaction and realize I have a choice not to fall into the whirlpool. The program is very caring and compassionate, a big void for me. I have reconnected with nature, and can appreciate things with 'raisin mind.'"

It seemed that our modified version of the 8-week MBCT course was being found helpful by participants who attended at least four classes. However, we realized we should treat these comments with some caution, as they were given during the last class, when the mindfulness teacher was in the room, and so might reflect participants' wish to praise or please the teacher. We could be firmer about the conclusions if the same pattern appeared in measures taken by assessors who did not know which treatment group participants belonged to, and from neurological measures that cannot be made to look good. So, what did these find?

At the beginning of the trial, there were no meaningful differences between those who received MBCT right away and those whose participation was delayed. But, while participants in the wait-list group drifted back toward depression during the waiting period, those who received MBCT right away remained stable on some measures and improved on others. Recall that all participants started the trial when in remission—that is, while feeling well—so we would not in fact expect improvement, but rather stability of this good mood.

On the BDI-II, MBCT significantly reduced residual symptoms of depression, while no change occurred for those on the waiting list. This effect on depression was also found for those participants with a diagnosis of bipolar disorder, and there were even stronger differences for the reduction in anxiety between MBCT and wait list in those with bipolar disorder (Williams et al., 2008). MBCT participants also reported significantly less discrepancy from their ideal self-guides after the classes than participants in the wait-list group, in large part because those on the waiting list tended if anything to move toward increased discrepancy (C. Crane et al., 2008). Similarly, in frontal α-asymmetry, the MBCT group retained a balanced profile, whereas in the waiting-list group significant shifts toward right-sided activation (reflecting avoidance mode) occurred (Barnhofer et al., 2007). Thus it seemed that MBCT did indeed offer these vulnerable patients some relief from depression and protection from increasingly negative patterns of response.

So, Who Benefited, and Who Did Not?

Note the statement that opens the previous section: MBCT was helpful "to participants who attended at least four classes." Unfortunately, this represented only about 70% of participants. That is, 30% of our participants failed to complete the course. Clearly this was not satisfactory, although in fact high rates of dropout are not unusual in psychological treatment research (Crane & Williams, 2010). Most of our dropouts occurred at the very beginning of the process—within the first few sessions and sometimes even before a single session had been attended.

In summary, we found positive results for those who attended at least half the classes. But our dropout rate was disturbing. Something had to be done. Could we identify psychological factors contributing to early dropout? And if so, could we intervene to reduce their impact and help people to stay the course? How could we adapt our early contact with participants so as to prepare them for challenges that might arise and to enhance engagement, motivation, and persistence?

Who Was Most Likely to Drop Out from MBCT?

Fortunately, we were able to use data from our cognitive measures to help us to identify those most likely to drop out from MBCT. We could also explore differences between the patterns of dropout in MBCT and in the wait-list group, so as to establish whether dropout was due to something both groups shared (e.g., preexisting history or clinical state), or whether there was something specific about dropout in relation to MBCT.

It turned out that we could predict with 90% certainty who was most likely to drop out of MBCT: those most prone to avoid their difficult experiences or get caught up in depressive rumination. What was particularly disappointing was that, at the outset, we had carefully measured the cognitive "signature" of suicidal depression—the collapse in problem-solving effectiveness when in mild, transient induced low mood. *All* the most vulnerable people on this measure left MBCT prematurely (Crane & Williams, 2010). Thus the people *most* likely to leave were exactly the people we were intending to help. We then looked to see if these factors predicted dropout from the trial overall (even in the control group). They did not. The conclusion was stark: *the most vulnerable patients at highest risk of suicide were the ones most likely to give up even before starting, or to leave the MBCT course in the very early stages.* We still did not know if MBCT would be helpful for the most vulnerable.

What could be done? We had a program which seemed to hold promise for people suffering recurrent suicidal depression—but only if they were able to engage with it in the first place, and to stay the course. Perhaps we could modify the precourse interview between teacher and participant so as to highlight potential challenges and better prepare patients to meet them. But first, we would need to consider what might make MBCT so intimidating a prospect for people, and to scrutinize closely our initial meetings with potential participants at greatest risk.

Obstacles to Engagement with MBCT

The findings from our pilot trial suggested that encounters with depressed mood, followed swiftly by getting caught up in self-defeating rumination and experiencing a collapse in problem-solving capacity, might well be contributing to participant withdrawal, often at an early stage. But this was not enough information. It did not give the "lived experience" of participants as they entered MBCT, and what factors meant they could not continue. So we asked our colleague Ann Hackmann, a clinical psychologist with many years' experience of working with the most vulnerable patients, to invite those who had dropped out to an interview in which they could talk openly about their experience. The results of her work suggested a number of factors that might stand in the way of engagement, and that could perhaps be addressed during entry to the trial. Most are familiar to mindfulness teachers: all are critical to take into account when those dropping out are the ones at highest risk. Here is what she found.

Making Time

> "Making the time was hard. Two hours is a lot out of an evening, and I had a long drive to get there and back too. It was tiring, at the end of the day."
>
> "I just couldn't do the practices every day–too much else on my plate. I felt really guilty."

In addition to eight weekly 2-hour classes, and perhaps a full day of guided meditation practice toward the end of the course, plus travel time, participants are invited to do up to 1 hour's home practice, 6 days out of seven, throughout the course. This is a substantial chunk of time to fit into a busy life, remembering that our participants were well when they attended, and often had significant work and family commitments to juggle too. When they were coping on a day-by-day basis, albeit with some difficulty, why would they wish to open themselves up to more distress?

People's life circumstances were not always easy. Some, for example, had difficult relationships with partners or family, some were experiencing financial difficulties, some suffering poor physical health, some overstretched and stressed by legitimate pressures (e.g., people with demanding, responsible jobs, and single parents with young children). Under such circumstances traveling to weekly classes and doing daily meditation practice, instead of being a source of nourishment and clarity, might become yet another thing that *had* to be done, another item on an already long list of burdensome tasks. Additionally, some had difficulty with taking time for themselves—it seemed selfish or self-indulgent to put themselves first in this way. Both of these issues would be more likely to emerge at times when mood was fragile.

Coming into Close Contact with Difficult Thoughts and Emotions

> *"Doing the course may have made it worse for me, by bringing things to the fore."*

> *"I expect it's necessary to get close to the difficult stuff, but I felt down as a result. I wonder if it's wise to keep dwelling on my depression."*

> *"It was hard to switch off afterward, if I was dealing with difficult stuff."*

We have already discussed the challenge presented by the central intention of the program: to learn to respond differently to painful thoughts and feelings, including depression and despair. In the past, participants may have devoted considerable effort and energy to protecting themselves from distress by avoiding and suppressing painful thoughts and feelings, or by trying to think their way out of trouble. It may feel as if these strategies are the only route to staying safe and resolving the difficulties they face (Watkins, 2008; Wells, 2009). The intention of the course is to give people an opportunity to learn new responses in relation to relatively benign everyday ups and downs. However, for our most vulnerable participants, the pilot trial told us that powerful negative thoughts and intense feelings might be readily triggered even by small downward shifts in mood. If then they slipped into ruminative brooding, or gave way to the natural urge to avoid something so aversive, what might otherwise be a transient state would likely both intensify and persist, perhaps confirming existing fears about the dangers of going anywhere near depression and the risk of relapse. These difficulties would be intensified at those times when, for whatever reason, mood dipped.

Expecting Too Much Too Soon

"It triggered lots of thoughts of failure."

"I thought, surely I should be getting somewhere by now?"

"You feel really enthusiastic to start with, and then something goes wrong, and you think, 'Why bother to go? There's no point.'"

Mindfulness meditation training is not an easy task. This can spark both self-judgment and judgment of the process. Depression in general and suicidality in particular are linked to a negative sense of self, often associated (as Beck's cognitive model of depression suggests) (Beck, Rush, Shaw, & Emery, 1979) with unreasonably high personal standards: "shoulds" such as perfectionism (O'Connor, O'Connor, O'Connor, Smallwood, & Miles, 2004), or the need always to please others, or to be in control (in short, discrepancy-based processing; O'Connor, O'Carroll, Ryan, & Smyth, 2012). These can come into operation in response to difficulties in home practice, just as they would in any other problem situation, giving rise to a pressure to "get it right," or to get immediate results, or (when the road is rocky) a sense of failure. Thus home practice itself can act as a mood induction procedure, if people do not appreciate it as a gradual learning process with natural obstacles and plateaus and recognize their reactions as old patterns of self-judgment turning up yet again.

Being Part of a Group

"Having to introduce myself at the beginning was very difficult"

"I prefer NOT too much sharing of personal issues—mine or those of others. It takes time to build trust, and I prefer only to do it with close friends."

> *"I find it very difficult to be in a group.*
> *I don't interact much, and I'm afraid I'm causing*
> *an atmosphere. I just wanted to run away."*

> *"I don't like being in a room*
> *with all these mentally ill people."*

The experience of being part of a group and sharing common experience is often a key element of participants' experiences, valued because it emphasizes common humanity and connectedness to others, which is the reverse of the sense of isolation often present in depression. However, for some participants, the idea of sharing experiences with a group of strangers was in itself intimidating. A few actually met diagnostic criteria for social phobia, with concerns about evaluation by others to the fore. Even where this was not the case, speaking out in front of a group is commonly experienced as anxiety-provoking, the more so when downward shifts in mood activate the urge for withdrawal that often accompanies depression.

Being the Odd One Out

> *"I felt uneasy, being the only man."*

> *"I did not fit in very well–I seemed to be more unwell*
> *than everyone else."*

> *"I felt really guilty, because I just seemed so cheerful*
> *compared to everyone else."*

The pilot trial told us that participants who dropped out of MBCT were significantly younger than those who continued. Initially, we thought this had to do with being young (perhaps not yet having sufficient experience of depression to be willing to take on the substantial home practice commitment?). It occurred to us, however, that this finding could simply be a reflection of the difference in age between younger participants and other members of the group. Most participants were in their 40s–60s. People could experience being the "odd one out" for a number of different reasons, as the comments above show.

It was clear that we had to do something that would keep vulnerable participants engaged with mindfulness from the earliest point in the process, yet give them the freedom to step away from it if it proved too difficult for them at this stage in their lives. And we could not wait until the first class. We needed to change what we did from the very first time we met prospective participants—the preclass interview.

Changing the Preclass Interview

The preclass interview has always been important for a number of reasons. Now we saw that it was absolutely critical for those participants at highest risk of suicide. Those who were most reactive were those most likely to drop out from a program that might otherwise offer them valuable opportunities for new learning. We will explore each of the issues we needed to address in turn. First, Table 6.1 identifies the main roles of the preclass interview.

As described above, the pilot trial gave us useful clues as to what might be important here. From its results, we could see clearly that the mood challenge task offered important confirmation about the signature characteristics of those most vulnerable. But it may also have activated old concerns at too early a stage. Was there another way of assessing risk of dropout? Indeed there was: those most likely to drop out were participants who scored highest on ruminative brooding and on a scale measuring avoidance of inner experience. These could be assessed without subjecting people to mood challenge. So we set up a system in which the course teacher would either be told by the assessor if the participant scored highly on rumination or avoidance, or would "listen out for" signs of both. We could then be alert to key signs of the intolerable despair and suicidality that signal the presence of "driven-doing mode," attempts to deal with intense pain that might then backfire, with tragic consequences. Teachers would then be prepared to take all necessary steps if concerned about a participant's safety.

In addition, they could prepare participants for other, more common or garden variety difficulties that might arise. They could, for example, be explicit about the substantial commitment of time required, and gently investigate what difficulties might arise in finding it. They would have some idea if the participant was likely to be an "odd one out," and could discuss how he or she might respond helpfully to this uncomfortable situation. They could warn participants

TABLE 6.1. The Role of the Preclass Interview

1. *Forging a working alliance between teacher and participant.* If the program is offered in a class format, it offers what may well be the only one-to-one opportunity for teacher and participant to speak in depth. Thus significant life events, issues, and concerns may be aired more fully than would normally happen in the class, where the focus is on learning and investigating closely the process of mindfulness meditation training as it unfolds, and where the participant may in any case feel less inclined to speak out. This is where rapport between teacher and participant can be established, and a trusting relationship formed.

2. *Understanding recurrent depression.* The interview allows the teacher to map out with the participant the trajectory of his or her depression, how and when it first began, what has happened since, how it is for him or her to be depressed (including especially talking openly about suicidal feelings). Through this discussion, understanding of the nature of recurrent depression (and suicidality) emerges from the mapping of personal experience. Participants can feel reassured that the teacher has an understanding of the condition and, rather than being disconcerted by talk of difficulty and despair, embodies calm steadiness and acceptance.

3. *Making the course rationale personally relevant.* Hearing participants' stories in some detail allows the rationale for MBCT to be shared in a way that is clearly directly relevant to each one's own experience of depression. So, for example, where rumination is key for a particular person, the idea of finding a different relationship to persistent thoughts might be emphasized. Where, on the other hand, the participant has an avoidant coping style, the value of approaching the difficult, and how the meditation practice helps, might take center stage.

4. *Identifying expectations and misapprehensions about mindfulness meditation.* By asking about previous experience of meditation (if any) and about expectations of what meditation means, misconceptions can helpfully be identified and corrected, for example, that the aim is to achieve a totally blank mind. The teacher can explain that the purpose of the practices is not to clear the mind but rather to become intimate with its workings, including those that create vulnerability to depression, although naturally it takes time and practice to know how best to deal with them skillfully.

5. *Outlining the practicalities of the course.* The basic practicalities of the course can be outlined, including dates and times (including a whole day of practice and follow-up meetings, if appropriate), what to bring, who else will be there, how to make contact if the participant cannot attend, and so on.

6. *Addressing potential difficulties and challenges.* Perhaps most importantly in the context of this chapter, the interview also offers an opportunity for the teacher to acknowledge that following this intensive program can be challenging, to speak openly about potential difficulties and anxieties, and to work with the participant to find possible solutions.

that meditation is not always pleasant and relaxing (it depends upon what turns up), and that experiencing difficulties is not in fact a sign that it is "not working." On the contrary, the greatest insights might emerge from the experience of difficulty. What makes the meditation practice difficult may also be the very thing that stands in the way of participants caring for themselves in other ways. So closely observing difficulties ("hindrances") could paradoxically be a valuable learning opportunity, and indeed directly related to people's prime intention in attending the course: to reduce the likelihood of relapse and recurrence.

This aspect of the interview includes an awkward and potentially discouraging element: no treatment of any kind, medical or psychological, can guarantee that a person who has experienced clinical depression will never experience it again. So the strongest position to be in is to accept that *it may revisit, given certain conditions, but that it is possible to learn to respond differently when it does, so that it may be less profound or last for a shorter time.* Even if depression returns, it may become possible to treat oneself gently and with compassion, as one might a good friend who is much loved, rather than adding to the burden of depression with self-criticism and hopelessness. In one way, this could be seen as something of a bleak prospect. But the essence is a hopeful message: "There is something you can do." Sensitively handled in the safe context of the interview, it may be helpfully realistic rather than demoralizing.

As we moved toward our major clinical trial, our sense of the importance of the preclass interview as a way of encouraging engagement and persistence increased. This is reflected in the fact that its format and function are described in some detail in the second edition of the MBCT manual, as they were not in the first (Segal et al., 2013; Ch. 6). Here we focus on elements of the process particularly intended to help the most vulnerable participants, those most likely to drop out.

The key change of emphasis in the preclass interview was to spend more time exploring with participants those aspects of engaging with the course that they might find difficult or challenging, and put these in the context of what they most wanted and hoped for (release from future depressions). We used the findings from the study of attrition from the pilot trial, and data more informally gathered from participants in early classes, as guides. Thus we hoped to encourage a sense that, though this might not be an easy journey, it would be worth staying the course, because MBCT would directly address the main reason why they were here.

We *extended the time allocation from one to 1.5 hours per participant,* so that there would be time to deal with information gathering, discussing the nature and form of the program, and (most importantly) reflecting on possible challenges and how they might best be met. The actual time for interviews varied, according, for example, to how easy participants found it to speak, how quick they were to grasp the nature of what they were embarking on, and so on. We devised a checklist of topics that it was important to address, and these were reinforced in a printed handout which participants took away at the end of the interview (they were also invited to contact the teacher if anything else that seemed important came to mind or if, once they got home, they felt unclear about anything). The key topics are detailed in Chapter 6 of the second edition of the MBCT manual (Segal et al., 2013), and outlined in Table 6.2.

Our Starting Point: "What Brings You Here?"

We begin by offering an opportunity for participants to tell their stories. We guide this process using open questions designed to help them to reflect on the course of their depression and its unique expression, and to be attentively and empathically heard. Thus teachers gather information on the particularities of *this* person's history, current symptom pattern, reactions to the recurrence of low mood, and understanding of how depression works, which will allow them to make discussion of the program's intentions and form personally relevant.

TABLE 6.2. Overview of the Preclass Interview

- "What brings you here?" How we understand recurrent depression.
- "How will mindfulness-based cognitive therapy be helpful to you?"
- Continuing to practice at home.
- Challenges that may show up when taking the MBCT course.
- The need for confidentiality.
- Practical arrangements.
- Concluding the interview.

Note. Based on Segal, Williams, and Teasdale (2013).

At the same time, the focused questions they ask, together with their attentive listening and empathic responses, reassure patients that they have an understanding of the condition, and can embody kindness and steadiness even in the face of revelations of early abuse, despair, and suicidality.

Understanding Depression

Ideally, discussion of the nature of vulnerability to depression (pre-existing cognitive patterns, and postepisode cognitive reactivity), and associated psycho-education, arises out of the patient's story, rather than being (as it were) an entirely separate item on the agenda. This process offers an opportunity to put unhelpful thinking, entanglement in ruminative brooding, and avoidance in context, to show how they are a natural part of the development and persistence of depression, and how recognizing them for what they are (rather than buying into them) opens up choices in how best to respond when depression visits once more.

Primary Vulnerability

Often it emerges that depression first occurred in the context of painful early experiences—in the family, in school, or in relation to broader social pressure and adversity (50% of our patients experienced their first episode during childhood or adolescence). These childhood experiences need not be openly abusive: for example, parents who are critical and perfectionistic on their child's behalf because they believe this is the best way to teach them to succeed in life, or a family that (almost absent-mindedly) fails to give the child a sense of intrinsic worth, can also leave an enduring negative sense of self, to which the child may respond with compensatory overdemanding standards. These in turn can then drive patterns such as feeling obliged to overperform at all times despite the personal cost, or being unable to assert needs, wants, opinions, and wishes (Beck et al., 1979). Such patterns may in themselves contribute to onset of episodes—for example, when someone who sets a premium of always performing 110% is unable to do so for some reason, and reacts with a sense of personal failure and with harsh self-criticism—which inevitably fuel low mood.

Postepisode Vulnerability

Here is where cognitive reactivity comes in, the growing strength of associations between different elements of depression, which means that if any one element is activated, even to a minimal degree, the others follow with increasing ease. So a perfectly ordinary, everyday dip in mood, such as anyone might experience when things are not going too well, would call up negative patterns of thought that would intensify the low mood, and readily slip into ruminative brooding or attempts to avoid or suppress. These attempts to short-circuit depression would then in fact increase the chances that it would deepen and persist. This was what we had seen in the pilot trial in our most vulnerable participants: those most likely to drop out of the program were also those whose capacity to problem-solve collapsed in the presence of mild, transitory low mood. The sequence is illustrated for one particular patient in Figure 6.1, drawn out as it was on the whiteboard in the class.

In the interests of beginning to cultivate the capacity to decenter from compelling thoughts and painful emotions, it was important to help participants to recognize that depression is not a sign of personal inadequacy or weakness but rather a normal human response to adversity and loss. Participants may also need to know that, episode by episode, depression becomes increasingly autonomous (the switch can be turned on, as it were, by a lighter and lighter pressure) so that in the end even trivial events and everyday shifts in mood can be enough to activate the system. This is an important realization for many people, whose reactions to experiencing depressed mood are compounded by feeling that this just doesn't make sense, nothing has happened to justify such a reaction, so it can only mean that there is something fundamentally wrong with them, and that there is nothing they can do about it (as shown in Figure 6.1).

> The increasing autonomy of recurrent depression—with each episode needing smaller triggers than the last—is an important realization for many people. Their reaction to depression is usually compounded by the feeling that "This just doesn't make sense" or "I have no reason to be depressed."
>
> Understanding a little of how depression affects the mind/brain can bring relief—"It's not my fault."

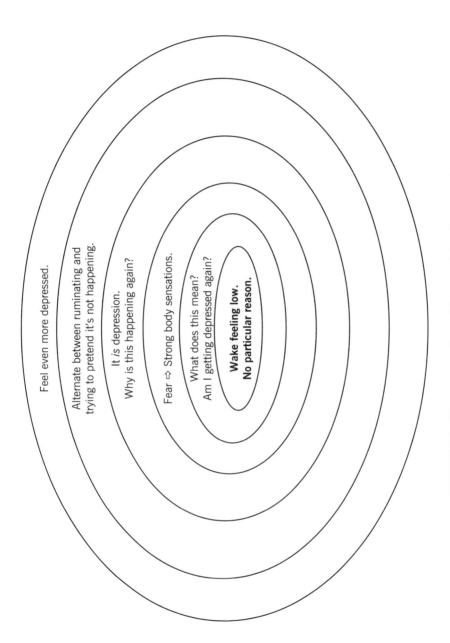

Feel even more depressed.

Alternate between ruminating and trying to pretend it's not happening.

It *is* depression. Why is this happening again?

Fear ⇨ Strong body sensations.

What does this mean? Am I getting depressed again?

Wake feeling low. No particular reason.

FIGURE 6.1. The process of cognitive reactivity: An example.

To facilitate understanding, we used the "tuning fork" diagram shown in Figure 6.2, personalizing it for each person by relating each element to their own experience, and proceeding as far as possible through inquiry rather than pure didactic teaching. What had they noticed about their thinking when depression was present? And what was the impact of gloomy, negative thinking on mood? (We may gently note the beginnings of a vicious circle here.) And what about negative thinking when they are well, or at least relatively well? Does it vanish, or is it more that it recedes into the background, that it is easier to dismiss or answer back? Could they imagine the pattern shown on the horizontal line extending back into the past, episode by episode, and the relationship between thinking and mood getting ever stronger and stronger? Of course they were well right now—otherwise they would not be taking part in the trial—but life being what it is, it was likely that at some point there would be a "flashpoint" for feeling down. It need not be anything dramatic—just some minor event, or even low mood turning up for no particular reason. If that happened, what would be the likely impact on their thoughts? And how might they then react? What would they do, in response to feeling low mood and negative patterns of thinking gearing up yet again? What thoughts would likely come to mind? About themselves? About their lives? About the future? What would be likely to happen then—might they just get caught up in the thoughts, going round and round (ruminative brooding)? Or

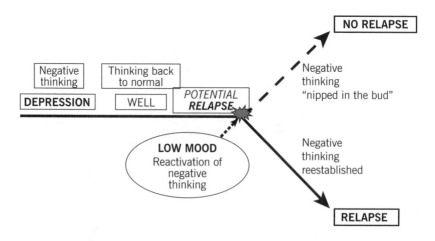

FIGURE 6.2. How do we understand recurrent depression?

might they try to ignore what was happening, or distract themselves (avoidance)? And what would be the consequences?

This would lead us to the fork in the diagram, the point where, if they were unable to identify what was happening, they might spiral down into depression. And thus we reach the purpose and intention of MBCT: to help participants refine their awareness of early warning signals of relapse, and to learn new ways of responding so that the slide into depression would be short-circuited. If people were concerned that they might miss these early warning signals, they could be reassured that it was possible to recognize the presence of depression and move to a new pattern of response at any point on the downward slope.

The Course: Purpose and Format

Just as hearing the patient's story and discussing the nature of depression offer opportunities to identify particular patterns of thought and behavior that may be instrumental in triggering and maintaining depression, so discussing the nature and intentions of MBCT offers an opportunity to be open about challenges participants may encounter during the program. Some of the most common issues are explored below.

It is important to be realistic about the extensive commitment that is needed to maintain home practice. How will participants make time for it in their everyday lives? Indeed, *can* they do so? If not, this may not be the right time to embark on the program. It is quite true that this is a substantial commitment, and of course participants may decide at the end of the course that this approach is not for them right now, perhaps never. However, they will not be in a sound position to make that decision wisely unless they have committed to making the investment in time and effort, opening up the possibility of seeing for themselves what the landscape of their lives might be if they could, even for a moment, trust that there was a different way of living their lives, one free from harsh judgment and unendurable suffering.

When asked about their previous experience of meditation, and their ideas of what it consists of, many people describe something rather different from what mindfulness meditation will offer. Some have tried some form of concentration meditation, where intense attention to a specific focus (a sound, a mantra, the breath, a candle flame), together with immediate dismissal of intruding thoughts, cultivates the capacity to concentrate deeply. Or perhaps they understand meditation as a form of relaxation, accompanied by visualizations. Either way, this is rather different from what they will encounter in MBCT. In particular, many other forms of meditation do not encourage growing familiarity with the workings of the mind, an open-hearted intimacy with what has been most toxic. This "willingness to experience" the difficult brings a clarity that is called "decentering" and this is central to mindfulness meditation. It means that (depending on what emerges) the practice may be anything but relaxing, and that rather than swiftly dismissing thoughts that arise, a moment is taken to acknowledge and welcome their presence, even if they are painful, before returning the attention to the intended point of focus (the breath, the body, sound, etc.). This learning in the first half of the course becomes the foundation for venturing intentionally into contact with difficulty in the second half, which is vital if participants are to learn how to respond with steadiness and kindness even to intense mental pain.

We learned that this was where it was vital to spend additional time. Given that it is usual for people to experience difficulties in carrying out the home practice, and to encounter difficult feelings as they meditate (perhaps feelings that they usually make efforts to avoid), we needed now to take time to explore reactions to this idea. How might they encourage themselves to take this challenging step? What will they do when they feel like giving up the course (as our research was telling us that they would)? What support might be helpful in the process, from the teacher, and also from people they know well and trust outside the class? What might be the advantages of allowing themselves to come closer to difficult thoughts and feelings? It may even be helpful to ask the participant what he or she might miss if all his or her meditations were peaceful and relaxing. What would he or she *not* learn? And how does that relate to his or her reasons for attending the class? We reminded them that the focus of the classes is on learning, rather than on revealing their personal history or in-depth exploration of problems in living—in other words this is an educational process, a class, not a therapy group. How does that strike them?

And they will be learning as part of a group. Might there be any difficulties for them there? Participants are often curious as to who else, and how many, will be present, so here is a chance for the teacher to note how much of the learning will come from one another, and to highlight the richness of the group experience, especially where the class contains many different people and personalities. This is also an opportunity to discuss with participants if we or they feel they might be "odd ones out" in any sense (e.g., age), and to inquire into how they might feel about that, and how nonetheless they might make the most of the experience.

Equally, speaking up in a group of strangers is a common human anxiety ("What will they think of me? Will I make a fool of myself? Will they like me?"), intensified if this is a person with significant social anxiety or social phobia. Here is where the teacher can emphasize that there is no requirement to speak out, and that respectful attentive presence is in itself a gift to other participants. In any case, whether in the large group, smaller groups, or pairs, whatever is said in the class is absolutely confidential and remains in the class. For some participants, contributing to the group became a sort of extended experiment, an opportunity to respond to fear in a different way, in the moment, as classes unfold.

Here too is an opportunity to acknowledge that, almost inevitably, there will be ups and downs during the 8 weeks—life events perhaps and, within the course itself, times of confusion and demoralization. This is not unusual, and need not be taken as a signal that MBCT is "not working." Changing the habitual patterns of mind and body that have accumulated over a lifetime can be a slow business. The seeds of the new need to be planted, exposed to the light, and watered for an extended period. The fact that they have not yet emerged from the ground is not a sign that they are not growing. Many participants smile in recognition when we talk of the constant (but unhelpful) urge we all have to dig up new seeds to see if they are taking root.

> Times of confusion and demoralization over the 8 weeks are not unusual, and need not be taken as a signal that MBCT is not working. Changing the habitual patterns of mind and body that have accumulated over a lifetime can seem slow, and no participant need struggle alone.

It is really useful for participants to realize that they are not alone when the going gets tough and particularly when they are tempted to give up. They are welcome, at any point, to contact the teacher between sessions, for a conversation face to face, or by telephone, or by e-mail. The teacher also lets them know that, if they are unable to attend and have not made contact, he or she will contact them to see if they are all right and to bring them up to date, and asks if that would be okay.

In addition, teachers need to be alert during classes for signs of difficulty, distress or struggle—not just during the class, but on arrival, during breaks, and at the point of departure—and when this happens to be willing to contact the participant to offer support. All our experience suggests that such sensitivity and caring in, around, and between sessions is valued rather than experienced as intrusive. When participants are potentially suicidal, this aspect of the process becomes even more important. During the preclass interview, the teacher needs to inquire openly whether this has been an aspect of depression for this person, and agree what will happen if it recurs. The top priority is the participant's safety and well-being. We have discussed this topic in detail in Chapter 5, but it is worth restating here some of the most important points.

An important step is, at some point in the preclass interview for those at risk of suicide, for both participant and teacher to *recognize and acknowledge the presence of suicidal feelings and thinking*, often in the form of powerful images. The teacher encourages the participant to *contact his or her family doctor, or if appropriate another professional* involved in his or her care if this becomes overwhelming. The teacher also needs to *clarify what will happen if the client is currently or becomes high risk, yet refuses to contact anyone*, which may involve a legal obligation to communicate with the family doctor or other professional on the participant's behalf. It has sometimes been assumed that one should not speak with people about suicidality, as it might put ideas into their heads. In fact, understanding it as part of the constellation of depression, and being willing to talk about it openly, in a matter-of-fact manner and with warmth and concern may be reassuring and create a sense of being held and secure in the vulnerable participant (Gould et al., 2005).

Concluding Remarks

We had extended MBCT to allow ourselves to focus on those at most risk of suicide, then piloted it to see if it was helpful. It was very helpful for those who stayed, but one in three had not managed to stay long enough to experience four or more sessions of the program. Those who dropped out were just the people whom we knew to be most vulnerable. These were the people who reported that when they became even a little depressed, they become avoidant, brooding about things, and we had found that under laboratory conditions their ability to solve problems collapsed. We had conducted qualitative interviews with those who dropped out in order to discover more about their experience. As a result of our quantitative and qualitative findings we had modified the preclass interview, allowing more time to discuss all the themes that had emerged from them. It was getting near the point that we would be ready to conduct a large randomized controlled trial to see if depression and suicidality might be reduced in this vulnerable group. We approached the trial feeling that we had made significant changes to the "gateway" into MBCT. But would it be enough? Would the changes we had made to encourage engagement and continued persistence be reflected in dropout rates for our clinical trial?

The answer was "yes." We shall report the full results of the trial itself in Chapter 18. But it is relevant to say now that, instead of the pilot trial dropout rate of 30% among our MBCT participants, in our large trial of 274 people only 7% failed to complete four or more sessions. We had found a way to explain the intentions of the course, and to engage and motivate people. Now we were ready to take the next step: to investigate the program itself and decide if we needed to make changes to what it contained and shifts of emphasis in how it might most helpfully be delivered. In the next sequence of chapters, we shall describe, session by session, what we did.

CHAPTER 7

Session 1:
Awareness and Automatic Pilot

Session-by-Session Descriptions: An Overview

After our pilot trial had revealed the critical importance of the preclass interview, we were ready to move on with the actual MBCT sessions. But we faced a crucial question: How could we best help people so vulnerable and at risk of suicide to remain steady and kind to themselves in the face of mental pain so intense that it feels intolerable? How could we help them to experience even *these* mind states as passing internal events, to which they could learn to respond with compassion, rather than reacting with avoidance or becoming entangled in rumination? We knew from the pilot trial that dropout and failure to engage were significant barriers to benefiting from MBCT's transformative potential. Making changes to the preclass interview was one part of tackling these barriers. Would this be enough—or should we also make changes to the protocol itself? On the basis of what we had discovered about vulnerability, this was what we decided to do. Because MBCT has been successfully manualized, it might be seen as fixed in stone. But, in fact, like all sound evidence-based therapeutic approaches, it is a living being, evolving in response to developments in theory, research, and practice. How much evolution was called for now?

In the next series of chapters, we describe what we discovered as we offered MBCT to those at high risk of suicide, and the specific (sometimes subtle) changes we made to the original 8-week program so that it might more readily meet the needs of these vulnerable participants. The changes included enhanced preparation for the stumbling blocks that might be encountered when attempting daily mindfulness practice at home (Sessions 1 and 2) and increased emphasis on mindful movement (Sessions 3 and 4); an extended focus on the mental pain of despair, as well as clarification of the nature and role of behavior intended to provide relief from painful thoughts and feelings, but in fact contributing to its persistence (Session 5); and extending the curriculum on cultivating awareness of personal relapse signatures and on how best to respond to these warning signs of self-destructive thoughts and feelings (Sessions 6–8).

Attending MBCT classes (like any other mindfulness intervention) invites insight into and familiarity with the workings of the mind and body, the shifting patterns of attention, the preoccupations, the coming and going of shades of emotion, the constantly changing landscape of sensations within the mind/body. For our vulnerable participants, even though at the time of the classes they were relatively well, this journey of exploration almost inevitably entailed encounters with difficulty—as indeed we now emphasized in our preclass interview. In MBCT, although systematic focused work on turning toward the difficult begins in Session 5—when meditation practices explicitly designed to help participants respond in new ways to painful material begin—difficulty and distress do not wait to emerge until this point is reached. On the contrary, mindfulness meditation can highlight distress right from the start, as it asks practitioners to become aware of their inner and outer worlds beginning with Session 1. As we shall see, even in the practice of eating a raisin can bring up unwanted thoughts, images, memories, feelings, and body sensations—the echoes of a deeper mental pain that is never far away.

So even in the meditation practices and psychoeducational elements of Sessions 1–4, repeated practice of the body scan, mindful movement, and sitting practices allow participants to notice again and again how readily the mind is pulled away from any intended point of focus, and how easily it is then seduced by the pull of negativity. Again and again, participants are invited to notice the wanderings of attention, to take a moment to acknowledge where it has gone (rather than brutally pulling it back), and then gently to return it to where they intend it to be. Even if it is never explicitly said by the teacher, this communicates an important message: you cannot stop the mind from wandering because that is what it is designed to do, but you may be able to exercise more choice in what happens next. You can consciously decide what to do when faced with the tendency to suppress this train of thought or this emotion, or to become entangled in thinking about it. Is it possible instead to see it as a mental event and release it? Choosing to let go, in turn, communicates another central message: no matter how compelling this train of thought is, it's okay to leave it be for now. You need not pursue it, or strive to avoid it, or believe it, or do what it says.

These early sessions also include cognitively oriented psychoeducational exercises designed to illuminate the relationship between thought and emotion, and in particular the role of negative thought patterns in precipitating and prolonging low mood ("Thoughts and Feelings" in Session 2; the Automatic Thoughts Questionnaire in Session 4). These build on the understanding of depressive relapse introduced in the preclass interview, and offer participants a more decentered view of automatic reactive patterns, a sense that they can (so to speak) stand a little to one side and observe the depression mechanism doing what it does without getting caught up in the moving machinery.

Through these complementary learning processes, the aim is for participants gradually to discover that it is possible to take their thoughts less personally, to know them for what they are: transient mental events, old and sometimes unkind and unhelpful habits of mind. Even if thoughts are compelling and charged with emotion, it does not follow that they are true, or integral to identity. So they can be greeted benignly ("Ah, here are thoughts about x or y") and allowed to come and go in their own time. This message, derived from repeated personal experience of mindfulness meditation, and highlighted through the process of inquiry, is foundational to responding to difficulty from a new perspective and with compassion. Let us now turn to Session One.

Session 1

The syllabus for Session 1, the intentions of each element, and associated home practices are summarized in Table 7.1.

TABLE 7.1. Week 1: Summary of Practices

Session theme	Practices and exercises	Skills learned	Insights supported by practices	Home practice
Awareness and automatic pilot	*Raisin exercise (Audio Track 2[a])*	To begin to experience the shift from "doing" mode to "being" mode. To experience the qualities of mindful attention.	Experiences can be richer if we pay full attention. Much of our everyday experience is missed because the mind is elsewhere.	*Mindfulness of everyday activities*
Aim: to explore how, on automatic pilot, it is easy to drift, unawares, into "driven-doing" mode and the ruminative thought patterns that can tip us back into depression. Habitual doing mode also robs us of our potential for living life more fully. We can transform our experience by *intentionally* paying attention to it in particular ways. We begin to practice stepping out of automatic pilot by paying attention, intentionally, mindfully, to eating: the sensations of the body, and aspects of everyday experience.	A meditation in which participants spend several minutes exploring the sensory features (sight, smell, taste, touch) of one raisin.			Participants choose a routine activity and attend to it mindfully.
	Body scan (Audio Track 3)	Sustained practice in engaging, disengaging, and shifting attention to different objects of awareness. Practice at returning the mind repeatedly to the intended object of concentration when it wanders.	Mind wandering is habitual. It is possible to develop greater awareness of bodily sensations (which may be associated with emotional states).	*Body scan*
	A guided meditation in which participants move their attention through the body attending to any sensations that arise in each area and breathing into each area.			Participants practice a body scan supported by Audio Track 3, on at least 6 days, noting their experiences.

[a]Audio recordings of the guided mindfulness meditation practices used in the MBCT program are available to readers for streaming or downloading at *www.guilford.com/williams6-materials*.

123

Reminding Participants of the Rationale for MBCT: Why Are We Here?

As we have already described in Chapter 6, we talk openly together during the preclass interview about the evidence that suicidal depression is a recurrent condition, triggered more and more easily as the number of episodes increases. In Session 1, after introductions have been made, and people have shared their first names and what they hope for from the course, we remind participants of the preclass interviews and the rationale for meeting together over the next 8 weeks. This includes highlighting the importance of recognizing and responding wisely to depression and hopelessness when they return, for this is the nature of the world in which these participants live. This powerful (and sometimes unwelcome) message, right at the start of the course, reflects the intention to keep these key issues explicit and central as we explore and discover mindfulness through meditation practices. Naturally, for participants who are well at this point, it can be challenging to bring to mind times when they have been depressed. Many have deliberately decided not to focus on these memories between episodes as far as possible, and may even have been hoping against hope that this time depression will not return. Yet unless these experiences are openly recognized, working with them (learning to be aware of their presence in the earliest stages and to respond effectively to them) is impossible.

Becoming Part of a Group

Groups can offer potent opportunities for participants to learn from each other. Yet learning to relate differently to oneself and others in a group context can be hard.

> Charles described his conviction that he must be the only person in the room to feel unsafe with others. After all, everyone else looked like they were doing fine in these first few minutes of the course. The introductions began, and one by one people named their anxieties about just being here in this group of people they didn't yet know, with similar experience to themselves. This helped him begin to wonder whether his belief that he was alone in feeling this way was accurate: perhaps he too looked less nervous than he felt. He also recognized his old familiar habit of believing he was different from others.

For many (like Charles) joining and being part of a group can trigger old anxieties and insecurities. Past problematic experiences in groups can emerge again. Humans have a strong need to belong and to be accepted and a common fear that this will not be so. All are vulnerable to fear of social isolation and exclusion. This natural fear may be even stronger in those who, as is often the case, see their depression as a sign of personal inadequacy. They rarely recognize the strength and courage it takes to live with it.

So, given their lifelong tendency to hide their experiences of suicidal depression, it is hardly surprising that some participants initially found being part of a group particularly challenging. The challenge showed itself in a variety of ways. Some were at first strongly reluctant to speak in front of the whole group. Others could not trust the group sufficiently to close their eyes during meditation practices, while others chose to sit in chairs rather than to lie down for early body scan practices, or lay in postures offering maximum protection, curled on their sides or wrapped in a blanket.

> One participant, Frances, described later in the course how terrified she was in the first class, feeling restlessness and irritation with everything about it, especially the sound of the bells. She needed to sit close to the door to feel safe enough to stay.

This sense of fear in the first class can be palpable and may be prolonged, as it is harder to settle in a group where many others feel similarly unsettled. Here the preclass interview can be helpful: many participants remarked that it eased their fears about joining a new group. They had already begun to develop a relationship with us, the teachers, and felt that we, and the intention of the classes, were trustworthy. McCown, Reibel, and Micozzi (2010) describe this role as *stewardship*, the teacher supporting and caring for the group, and thus creating a safe space where learning can arise. Participants begin to "raise their heads"—to observe others with similar fears, behaving in ways that reflect their own inner experience. This can be a revelation:

> Daphne said, with surprise, that hearing others in the group saying unkind things about themselves, when they so clearly didn't deserve this, really helped her acknowledge her own patterns of self-judgment.

Watching this thinking and behavior in the others gave her the perspective to "decenter" and see her own pattern clearly.

It is even more important than with other classes that the most vulnerable participants are repeatedly given permission to care for themselves, clearly and in a variety of ways, starting with the preclass interview. They are reminded they can choose how much to participate. They are encouraged to take care of themselves, for example, by having a drink when needed, taking comfort breaks, wearing layered comfortable clothing, and so on. Confidentiality, ground rules, and safety information are given in the initial interview, and repeated in Session 1, both verbally and in written form. These elements, along with the qualities consistently embodied by the teacher of warmth, patience, kindness, and acceptance communicate a sense of welcome, respect, self-care, and safety.

Raisin Exercise

The raisin exercise (Audio Track 2), the first meditation practice of the course, invites people to explore this small object as if for the first time. All the senses are used to explore the raisin and discover its characteristics. This small, unassuming object that many of us eat on a regular basis (perhaps mixed with nuts or in cereal) can turn out to be undiscovered territory, rarely even registered in the rush of life.

Most mindfulness teachers recognize that this simple eating meditation can begin to hint at a number of really important discoveries. Many participants are struck by the rich detail they discover by slowing down and paying attention, the pleasure of attending fully to encountering just one raisin, or the surprise at discovering that it may make a noise when gently moved between finger and thumb. The contrast between this careful attentiveness and heedlessly rushing past experiences, carried by the stream of life's busyness, is generally felt and easily named within the group.

In the classes for people with suicidal depression a wide range of experiences were reported. Many people described very similar positive experiences and reactions to those in other groups, but sometimes their experiences were more intense and in some cases much more negative. Some people described the raisin as "revolting" or "disgusting." It reminded them of something they wouldn't eat—insects or animal droppings. Some could not bring the raisin closer to their mouths than arm's-length, let alone explore and taste it. A bowl to collect "reject raisins" and wipes to remove the "unpleasant stickiness" remaining on fingers was sometimes needed. In one particular group, with 12 participants, half were unable to bring a single raisin to their mouths.

Such powerfully aversive reactions can be disconcerting for teachers, especially if (albeit implicitly) they have been expecting a more positive response. The saving grace is that, just as the instructions for the later practice of sitting with the difficult (Session 5) suggest: "Whatever it is, it's okay." There is as much learning to be had in the negative as there is in the positive—if not more—provided the teacher can respond, even-handedly, with the same embodied openness, interest, warmth, attentiveness, and willingness to explore. After all, here, early in the very first class, is a demonstration of the impact on body and mind of how things are perceived, the effect of labeling and associating present experience with the past, powerful reactivity to the unpleasant, with immediate urges to avoid—all arising from one short practice! Thus, for some participants at least, reactions to difficulty and aversion are immediately available to awareness—and this, of course, is the heart of the program, precisely what it is designed to address. For a teacher to conclude that the raisin practice "went badly" because of participants' aversive reactions would be like a physician concluding that listening to someone's chest through a stethoscope had gone badly because he or she had detected a sound that signaled the origin of a problem.

If the first participants to speak are those whose reactions were powerfully negative, it may be difficult for others to share their experiences, especially at this early stage where they have not as yet got to know one another. The reverse is also true—if initial reactions are strongly positive, then it may be hard for those whose experience was aversive to speak. So it is always worth asking: "Did anyone have a different kind of experience?"

Teaching when so great a range of experience is revealed underlined the importance for teachers of understanding clearly not only the intentions underlying the curriculum of *this* class, but also of later classes and how learning unfolds over the whole program, for example, through the thoughts and feelings exercise in Session 2 ("Walking Down the Street") or when working with the body's limits in Session 3's mindful movement practices (see below). However, a word of caution is due here: The curriculum is structured in order to unfold progressively, and we found that care needed to be taken not to allow the learning from later classes to be introduced too early (e.g., exploring too extensively how the mind interprets reality, or speaking of the need to "turn toward" a difficulty, when these topics will be explored in Sessions 2 and 5, respectively). This is balanced by the teacher's being responsive to what the group are experiencing right now:

> "Thank you so much for all your comments. Isn't it interesting how the same little object can bring out such different experiences in each of us? We all noticed different things about it. Everyone found that past experience was also right here with us as we looked at the raisin—memories of Christmas, or reminding us of things we knew such as animal droppings. We saw how much our perception of it and the thoughts we had about it influenced what happened then; whether we chose to explore it more closely or to keep it at a distance. Some of the ways that we approach life generally arose right here as we met these raisins!"

Body Scan

The body scan (Audio Track 3) can be challenging in many ways. Simply stilling the body for 30–40 minutes in the midst of a frantic pattern of living is by no means easy. In our busy world, relaxing is closely associated with falling asleep, and being alert with hypervigilance. Here we are inviting participants to explore the rarely trodden "middle path" of relaxed wakefulness. It is not easy. Immediately feeling like falling asleep, being constantly distracted by the "to do list" in the mind, becoming aware of the body *at all* after years of habitually discounting its messages—all these are common challenges presented by the body scan. Some participants have associations with past experience of progressive relaxation training and find it difficult to understand this practice as one where there is no required outcome. Some, of course, love the practice and welcome the opportunity to let go of driven-doing and simply be.

For our participants with a history of adversity, the Body Scan meant tuning into a wide range of experiences that were (at the very least) not as they wished, and maybe even threatening. The invitation to lie down in a strange place with people they hardly knew, paying attention to a body that they spent little time connected to in any positive way, was frequently challenging. Concerns about their ability to do this well/properly—to access sufficient sensory experiences, to focus attention, or to stay awake—often revealed a rich source of habitual patterns of reactivity. In a group where the experience of childhood abuse or trauma was frequent, the invitation to spend time, in a group of relative strangers, waking up to sensations in parts of the body associated with traumatic memories might seem particularly difficult or inappropriate. For this reason, we ensured that participants understood that it was okay for them to decide for themselves whether to take part or not, to sit or lie, to open or close their eyes, to choose where to focus their awareness (e.g., on the breath, the body as a whole, the floor or chair supporting them) if parts of the body were especially challenging. With this evidence of care and respect, the invitation was more readily accepted.

One participant, Anabel, was irritated with the practice because it had been "much too long." Lower back pain, which she knew well but generally managed to distract herself from, had been present throughout. During the enquiry she was angry and sat with her arms folded.

ANABEL: That was awful!

TEACHER: What was it that told you that, Anabel?

ANABEL: I haven't had that much pain in my back for ages. Lying down like that made it much worse. Why did it have to take *so* long?!

TEACHER: So, lots of irritation here right now? (*Anabel nods and unfolds her arms.*) And how is your back pain now?

ANABEL: Oh, it's gone now but it was awful.

(*There is a pause, an acknowledgment of this realization.*)

TEACHER: Would it be okay to ask a bit about the pain during the practice? (*Anabel agrees.*) I wonder when you first noticed it?

ANABEL: It first got difficult when I was supposed to be on my right knee.

TEACHER: But no pain before then? (*Anabel pauses as she reflects back and shakes her head looking a bit surprised.*) So where did you notice pain first?

ANABEL: (*Thinks for a moment or two.*) My tailbone started to be painful.

TEACHER: I wonder if you can say anything about what told you this was painful?

ANABEL: (*another pause*) It was tight.

TEACHER: Whereabouts? Did it cover a big part of your back?

ANABEL: No, just the bottom of my spine where it touched the floor.

TEACHER: You're clenching your fist just now, was that how it felt? (*Anabel nods.*) Were there any other sensations that you noticed that went along with the tightness?

ANABEL: No, but I started to get worried. I wanted to move but I didn't want to disturb anyone.

TEACHER: So, worry and thoughts about wanting to move? Did you notice anything happening in your body as these were there?

ANABEL: (*thinking for a few moments*) Yes, my chest started to feel tight too and I noticed it was harder to breathe.

TEACHER: And what happened then?

ANABEL: I wanted to move even more!

The teacher went on explicitly to acknowledge and welcome the detail in how Anabel noticed her experience and her contribution to the group. Then she moved back to working with the whole group, reflecting on this process of noticing whatever arises, and learning to recognize how mind and body interrelate, how, for example, the experience of pain can be transformed into suffering by the mind's reactivity: "I wanted to move but I didn't want to disturb anyone." Here is a microexample of entrapment, and we can see how quickly it can escalate into something much larger.

In this situation, choices and permissions were restated, so that the class could understand clearly that there is no prohibition on moving, when this feels the wisest option—even if it involves making some noise. The teacher might close the discussion with a light touch: noise might even be a welcome reminder to be awake for some people! As Anabel concluded, "Yes, I might move next time, but maybe if I remember I can it won't feel so bad and I will be able to concentrate on the practice."

Notice what has happened here. It would be easy for any teacher to be thrown off course by Anabel's unpleasant experience and her body language. However, the teacher (all too aware of some contraction in her own body as she heard Anabel's experience) took a moment to acknowledge this inwardly. So she was able to remain warmly open about what had happened, feeling curious rather than offering justifications or apologies. At a gentle but steady pace, she invited Anabel to explore and name the direct experience, dropping below the conceptual label ("pain") to the actual sensation of tightening, like the clenched fist.

Many possibilities arise in any inquiry process. The teacher here could have explored the experience of wanting to move away from the pain, or the thoughts about not upsetting others, or alternatively she could have explored what was also "right" about her experience of the practice. Understanding the intention of the practice at this point in the course guides the teacher in choosing which avenue to explore.

Setting Up Home Practice: Allowing Time to Prepare for Barriers

We knew from our early investigations that difficulty with regular mindfulness meditation practice was a common barrier to engagement. After Session 1, home practice consists of the 40-minute body scan (6 days out of seven), and daily "everyday mindfulness." This means bringing "raisin mind"—the same quality of sustained attention that had been experienced when eating one or two raisins in the first class—to the same routine activity each day, simple actions (like making a cup of coffee or taking a shower) that might normally be done on automatic pilot, with the mind elsewhere. Long formal practices and short everyday mindfulness practices present different challenges. The body scan takes a substantial amount of time, and may involve unpleasant experiences such as boredom, irritation, sleepiness, aches, and pains. Everyday mindfulness (such as attending to routine activities) takes very little "clock time," but you have to remember to do it, and this can be an added challenge for those who are likely to be plunged into despair by the thought that they are failing to do what they have been "told" to do.

Toward the end of Session 1, just as in the preclass interview, we openly acknowledged that these stumbling blocks might arise:

> TEACHER: So that's the home practice for this week—the body scan meditation, bringing "raisin mind" to the same routine activity every day, and exploring mindful eating. Let's take a few minutes to consider how it will be to have this daily commitment—it may not sound too difficult sitting here now, but when it comes to actually doing it, things may look rather different! For some people, just finding the time is a real problem. Or it could be that other things will come up and get in your way. Can anyone think of anything that might make doing regular home practice difficult?
>
> JO: Well, this week I'll have loads of work to do for my boss. He's under pressure himself and really getting at me. I don't know how I'll find the time.
>
> SALLY: My partner's away this week, and I have three children to take care of on my own.
>
> TEACHER: Thank you—these are really good examples of possible stumbling blocks. Problems and pressures like these could make it hard for you to do the practice. So let's take a few minutes to talk together in pairs, and help each other to identify what might get in your way. See if you can you help each other find ways to work with the difficulties that might turn up.

This opportunity to reflect and think ahead in pairs worked well, partly because it acknowledges the challenges from the outset, and partly because it allows the teacher to revisit such "barriers" during the home practice review in Week 2, to check in and see which of these actually happened, and whether there were new ones that had not been anticipated. This way of setting up home practice in Week 1 is now incorporated into the second edition of *Mindfulness-Based Cognitive Therapy for Depression* (see Segal et al., 2013, p. 129).

External pressures like the demands of work and the needs of a young family can be especially difficult to see a way through. There can be more subtle internal barriers too, for example, doubts and reservations about the program (e.g., "This looks like a lot of hard work. How can I be sure it'll work?"); emotional or physical states (e.g., a dip in mood, increased anxiety, or a feeling of fatigue); or habitual attitudes (e.g., "I must fulfill all my obligations before I take time for myself" or "I don't deserve this"). The discussion in pairs and the inquiry that follows allow participants to discover that they are not alone, and by hearing what others say they may tune into barriers they themselves had not yet identified, and perhaps begin to see that stumbling blocks to regular practice are part of a bigger pattern. The teacher's interest and acceptance encourages them to become curious about what might turn up. The teacher might close the discussion by drawing these threads together:

TEACHER: So, what did you notice from your discussions?

LEYLA: Well, it seems like pretty much everybody is going to have things getting in their way! (*laughter in the group*)

TEACHER: Yes, it does, doesn't it? Absolutely. Thank you. It's completely normal to run across stumbling blocks when we try to fulfill our intentions—things turn up that get in our way. Actually, not only is it completely normal, it's potentially a really valuable opportunity to learn more about what makes it hard to care for yourself in a much more general sense. Did anyone notice a stumbling block that might come up this week that also turns up in other situations?

JO: Well, I know I'm not good at putting my own needs first, even when it's really important. I always feel I have to do everything for everyone else first. (*nods from other participants*)

TEACHER: Thanks—and it looks like other people recognize that one? So perhaps the thing is to accept that stumbling blocks may turn up, so we can be alert for them, and observe them closely. What exactly is this getting in my way? Is it familiar? How can I best help myself to continue with the practice? Then next week we'll talk together about what happened, and what actually turned up. Was it what you predicted? Or something else?

LEYLA: Could be interesting!

TEACHER: (*smiling*) It could indeed.

In a sense, stumbling blocks are not the problem—they are a normal part of trying to pursue regular commitments amid the hustle and bustle of everyday life. What is important is not their presence, but rather how participants respond to them. If they can be recognized and approached with curiosity and interest (rather than viewed as an insuperable barrier or sign of failure), they offer valuable learning, opportunities to identify recurring situations and patterns of mind that regularly make life difficult.

> What is important is not so much that difficulties with practice arise, but rather what happens next. If difficulty is followed by self-judgment and giving up, then little learning is possible. If difficulty is greeted with recognition, acceptance, interest, and curiosity, then it can become the beginning of the transformation of despair.

Concluding Remarks

By the end of the first session, participants have already encountered key elements of the program. They have experienced two practices (the raisin and the body scan) which embody essential elements of mindfulness: precise, kindly awareness of the body, and openness to the richness of everyday experience—a direct antidote to automatic pilot and the busy "doing" mind. They have discovered that cultivating mindfulness will probably not be easy, but that difficulty itself is a rich source of new learning. They have met one another, and begun the process of realizing that depression happens to all sorts of people, and beginnings of an intimation that perhaps it is not after all a sign of weakness or inadequacy. And through the embodiment of the teacher, they have experienced a stance of kindly acceptance and compassion, a stance radically different from their own self-judgments.

CHAPTER 8

Session 2:
Living in Our Heads

In the home practice following Session 1, the body scan and routine activities have been assigned to begin to cultivate participants' skills in two areas of learning and growth: how to recognize/step out of automatic pilot and how intentionally to focus sustained attention in a single place. Session 2 gives the chance to revisit these themes many times.

In the original MBCT program, Session 2 was called "Dealing with Barriers." Its title reflected the discovery that, for most participants, this is a time when their attempts at home practice have revealed many issues and challenges that need to be addressed. The barriers were highlighted as important, first, because they can be demotivating if not seen as things that can be worked with; second, because they provide a golden opportunity to see, writ large, many examples of the doing mode of mind in action. In our continuing work with MBCT, however, it became clear that underneath the barriers, something else was going on that needed to be made explicit: overreliance on the aspect of "doing" that we call "conceptual mind" (see Chapter 2, Figure 2.1). In Session 2, the body scan is revisited, but now the teacher has the chance to fold another theme into the mix: inviting participants to become aware of how much of the time life can be lived in the head rather than directly through the senses, without awareness of the consequences.

Session 2

The syllabus, the intentions of each element, and associated home practices are summarized in Table 8.1.

Revisiting the Body Scan

The body scan practice (Audio Track 3) at the start of the class and the inquiry that follows can bring up many different sorts of issues that present choices to the teacher. Especially where aversive reactions are present, the invitation to be attentive to experience, whatever it is, long enough to know it better and see how it unfolds moment by moment is new to many. Equally, although we do not use these words, the distinction between attunement to pure sensation (experiential processing), as opposed to "thinking about" sensation (conceptual processing), can still be puzzling at this point.

The themes highlighted in the Session 1 and Session 2 body scans might be quite different from each other. Although participants have been practicing the body scan at home during the week, it is important to focus specifically on investigating *this* practice, rather than merging the discussion with the home practice review. This offers participants practice in focusing on *specific* experiences ("What is here, right now, in this particular moment?"), rather than inviting generalization to the narrative of the whole week. Once again, this invites direct experiencing rather than conceptual processing. We communicate clearly from the beginning of the course that we welcome all sorts of experiences, including difficult ones, fully open to exploring whatever arises with warm friendliness and interest. But in order to do so, we need to stay close to *this* experience, right now.

Home Practice Review

It is rare for participants in mindfulness courses to have completed all the home practices easily, without encountering at the least discomfort or boredom. People may be reluctant to "confess" to these difficulties initially. The importance of exploring the *process* of working with the intention to practice at home, rather than *doing* it successfully ("getting it right"), is yet to be felt and understood. The idea of home *practice*

TABLE 8.1. Week 2: Summary of Practices

Session theme	Practices and exercises	Skills learned	Insights supported by practices	Home practice
Living in our heads Aim: To provide an opportunity to explore a new way of knowing. In doing mode we "know about" our experience only indirectly, conceptually, through thought. We easily get lost in rumination and worry. In mindfulness we know directly, intuitively—"experientially." Experiential knowing is a way to be aware of unpleasant experiences without getting lost in rumination.	*Body scan (Audio Track 3[a])* As above. *Thoughts and feelings exercise* Participants imagine an ambiguous scenario (not being noticed by an acquaintance) and explore their reactions to such an event, as well as how these might vary as a function of mood.	To observe mind wandering, to practice letting go of thoughts and bringing attention repeatedly back to the intended object. To begin to reflect on the associations between thoughts, feelings, body sensations, and behaviors from a metacognitive perspective.	We have a tendency to judge our experiences as pleasant or unpleasant, to avoid unpleasant experiences and seek those that are pleasant. This triggers "thinking about" experience rather than staying with direct experience itself. Our interpretation of events (which may itself be influenced by mood state) influences subsequent emotions, cognitions, bodily sensations, and behaviors.	*Body scan* Participants practice a body scan supported by Audio Track 3 on at least 6 days, noting their experiences. *Noticing pleasant events* Participants are asked to notice events or moments they experience as pleasant and observe the thoughts, feelings, and bodily sensations that arise on these occasions.

[a]Audio recordings of the guided mindfulness meditation practices used in the MBCT program are available to readers for streaming or downloading at *www.guilford.com/williams6-materials.*

may rouse resonances of earlier experiences of home*work* (with all the automatic reactions this word brings from schooldays). There may be reluctance to talk about home practice because of the sense of shame in having failed to do the required tasks. Old habits of thinking about the "need to achieve" and "to do well at all tasks" may show themselves.

As we noted earlier, this was why in Session 1 we offered a more explicit focus on obstacles to practice, and devoted time in Session 2 to reviewing participants' actual experiences. The intentional focus on difficulty is balanced by acknowledging experiences that have been valued and welcomed. Once again, whatever it is, it's okay. All experiences are met by the teacher with warmth, gentle curiosity, and acceptance.

TEACHER: Let's move on to discuss the home practice. I'm interested to hear what your experience was.

ADAM: I found it really difficult to get through the body scan. I found I got very tense about it, and in the end I didn't want to do it at all.

TEACHER: Thanks, Adam. We spent a little time last week thinking about what difficulties might get in your way—and it sounds like this was a really tough one for you?

ADAM: Yes, it was. And then of course I felt bad—what's the point of coming if I can't even get through the first week?

TEACHER: Sounds like that was really discouraging. (*Adam nods.*) Let me just ask, (*turning to group*) did anyone else have difficulty doing the practice?

SEVERAL PARTICIPANTS: Yes!

TEACHER: This is really important to notice. Practically everybody who begins intensive training in meditation—which is what this is—comes across stumbling blocks at some point. So working out how to respond to them is really important. (*to Adam*) With that in mind, would it be okay to look more closely at what happened for you?

ADAM: Okay.

TEACHER: Was this a difficulty you had predicted last week? (*Adam shakes his head.*) So when did you first notice it?

ADAM: The second time I did the body scan.

TEACHER: At any particular point?

ADAM: I suddenly realized we were on the right foot, and I'd completely missed most of the left leg.

TEACHER: And what was your reaction when you noticed that?

ADAM: I thought "We've hardly started, but I'm already getting it wrong." I felt really disappointed in myself. I should be able to do better than that.

TEACHER: Really disappointed that you were getting it wrong. And then?

ADAM: I made myself go on, but I couldn't concentrate and I got really tense. And the next day I was completely on edge all the time, and I could hardly focus at all.

TEACHER: Where was your mind while that was going on?

ADAM: Same stuff really, beating myself up for getting it wrong.

TEACHER: And is that something familiar to you, beating yourself up?

ADAM: Too right!

TEACHER: So there's this sense that you have to "get it right," and as soon as something doesn't go as it should, you're criticizing yourself and feeling bad, and then of course you just want to forget all about it, what's the point? (*to Adam*) Is that right?

ADAM: Yes.

TEACHER: Thank you for describing this so well. Does this experience ring bells for anyone else? (*some nods*) What you've told us about is really valuable, you know, because seeing more clearly how we react when things get difficult, and learning how to respond to all of this, is an important part of these classes, for everyone. So here's an opportunity to explore, to see if it's possible when the practice is hard to take a moment to notice what's going on. What exactly is the stumbling block? Is it perhaps an old pattern of yours, like "I must get it right or I'm a complete failure"? It could be lots of things. What you're being invited to do here is notice that an old pattern has turned up again, and, for now, see if it's possible to acknowledge it's here, and then, as best you can, escort your mind back to the intended focus [the right foot or whatever]? (*to Adam*) Might you be willing to explore that possibility?

ADAM: I'll give it a go.

TEACHER: It's hard though, isn't it? At the moment, just having the courage to persist with it when everything inside you is screaming "This is no good" is amazing—thank you. Did anyone else have difficulty?

ROBERT: I was like Adam, I planned to do it and kept telling myself that I'd made the commitment to doing the homework and it was pointless coming to the classes if I don't practice at home but I just couldn't get myself to do it some days.

TEACHER: Thanks, Robert. It is really helpful to explore what happens for each of us with home practice. I expect you are speaking for lots of people here as it can be difficult to get ourselves to practice. Lots of resistance can materialize!

ISABEL: I put the CD on but fell asleep almost immediately. I felt really guilty about not doing it properly. (*Pauses a moment or two.*) I was really worried about saying anything today.

TEACHER: Thank you so much for having the courage to say this, Isabel. I'm sure you aren't the only one to have slept! (*Looks around the room and several people are nodding and acknowledging that they slept too, and Isabel looks relieved.*) So many times in our lives we do things to get somewhere particular or to do it well, don't we? What we're doing in these classes is quite different. We are practicing simply to learn to notice clearly our experience. So if we're sleepy, we just notice sleepiness.

The teacher continues to explore the group's various experiences of sleepiness, turning toward this unwanted experience with interest and friendliness. The group may find many types of sleepiness and thoughts and emotions arising from this. Some are recognizable to the whole group, some are individual reactions. The atmosphere in the class now has shifted from the embarrassed silence at the start of the home practice inquiry to more curiosity-driven conversation, and as a result participants are feeling much safer in sharing their experiences, even if they have been negative.

ZOE: I found it so difficult to lie still! I was fidgeting and squirming right through it.

TEACHER: So how did you work with this restlessness, Zoe?

And later:

GEORGE: My mind was all over the place! I lost about half of my body each practice, being off with some thought or other.

TEACHER: Ah, the body scan can offer us a good way of realizing how much of the time our attention is here or elsewhere, can't it? Did you notice some of the places your mind went to?

The willingness to explore with friendly curiosity experiences that might otherwise be seen as shameful or proof of failure is a radical shift for many. Of course the teacher in this situation could have chosen to focus on many different aspects of different participants' experiences, but the intention to explore without judgment or offering a solution is critical.

Notice what has happened here. What may be disconcerting and demotivating if unexpected and unprepared for can instead be understood by participants as a normal part of learning something new and sometimes difficult. Gradually participants may come to see that a stumbling block, and the demoralization or shame that it can bring in its wake, might become a valuable opportunity for exploration and insight. What's going on here? Is this a pattern? Where else in life can it be seen? How might I best respond to it when next it arises? Whatever happens, whether participants do the practice or not, whether it "works" or not, if they attend carefully to their experience, they might discover something of value about their lives and the workings of the mind.

Walking Down the Street

This exercise is designed to help participants explore how immediate interpretations shape emotional responses, how these are expressed in the body, and how they can lead to actions (or urges to act). We offer a simple scenario that is open to multiple interpretations:

"Imagine you are walking down the street, and coming the other way you see someone you know. You wave and smile, but he or she passes by without acknowledging you. How do you react? What thoughts come to mind? How do you feel [emotions, body sensations]?"

Participants are invited to share their experiences. Some are quick to think that the person who didn't wave just didn't see them. They may experience no particular emotional response, or perhaps something mildly positive (e.g., amusement), or perhaps a brief reactivity that passes quickly. On the other hand, the imagined situation could be taken in a very different way, for example, as a sign that you have offended the other person, or that he or she is deliberately ignoring you. These immediate interpretations can then spark painful memories, and inquiring may reveal that what has come to mind here, in a purely imagined scenario, represents an old and perhaps distressing pattern that has been present again and again, perhaps for many years. For those with repeated experience of suicidal depression, if this were a real situation, even a small amount of low mood might then trigger the cascade of hopelessness, rumination, and collapse of problem solving that we had shown to be central to vulnerability. Thus what might seem an everyday occurrence, open to interpretation, might with our most vulnerable participants offer a fast track to low mood, catastrophic thinking, and even suicidal thoughts.

So the messages communicated by this simple exercise may have immediate relevance, albeit implicit, to the processes at the root of vulnerability. First, it is possible and safe to begin to turn toward even difficult experiences, to explore them with curiosity, and so to discover the workings of the mind. Second, when we do so, we may discover that whatever happens can be seen from many perspectives, and perspective shapes what happens next. Third, experiences that may feel wholly idiosyncratic at one level may in fact be shared at another. The group experience offers a broader context in which common reactions may be acknowledged. It's not just me! So develops a growing sense of safety and companionship, and the group become a place where painful experiences may be recognized and named.

Pleasant Experiences Diary

> TEACHER: So how would it be if we allowed ourselves to be in touch with the range of pleasant experiences already present in our lives?
>
> PARTICIPANT: That sounds nice!

In mindfulness courses for participants who are not so vulnerable, the invitation to notice and record a pleasant experience each day is often welcomed. But for people with a history of depression, and especially suicidal depression, turning toward pleasant experience is not always welcome, easy, or experienced as mood-enhancing, as the examples below show:

- Sharon, on hearing about this home practice, said simply, "There won't be anything to record."

Note that the group are currently well as they attend the course, not depressed at this point. Some welcome it but then report back the following week:

- Mary: "When I did notice the lovely taste of the first sip of tea, I then noticed I was telling myself I was lazy to stay in bed to drink the tea! "

> Often, a range of *kill-joy* thoughts come up. Participants say they have many thoughts about *not deserving* pleasant experiences or *others being more worthy* of this, or sadness that *these experiences wouldn't last.*

- Jonathon: "I was sitting watching the sun setting over the sea and then suddenly I felt a rush of sad feelings. What a waste to have missed all these moments in my life!"

In setting up the home practice, and in reviewing it the following week, the aim is to use the diary of pleasant experiences to clarify what is actually arising: in particular, how do any of us know what is pleasant, directly? The aim of the practice is to help people see for themselves (and not because anyone else has told them) that all such experiences are multifaceted when explored in close detail—amalgams of thoughts, body sensations, emotions, and behaviors or urges. Seeing and feeling more clearly in this way brings new perspectives.

Session 2 ends with a short 5–10 minute sitting, in which participants are invited to bring the same quality of attention they cultivated in the body scan to the sensations of the breath (see Teasdale et al., 2014, Audio Track 4). Part of the home practice will be to do such a sitting with breath practice each day, as well as the body scan and bringing "raisin mind" to a different routine activity.

Concluding Remarks

Session 2, returning to the body scan, reveals how common the struggle to "get it right" may be, and how it takes us away from immediate experience. For the first time, a more explicitly cognitive element of the program is introduced to highlight the influence of habitual thought patterns on emotion, body sensation, and behavior. Through this exercise, participants often realize that they are not alone in self-blame and anticipating rejection; other people experience these painful thoughts too. This careful dissection of different elements of experience is then carried into everyday life, through the home practice focus on pleasant everyday experiences.

CHAPTER 9

Session 3:
Gathering the Scattered Mind

Session 3

Returning to the present moment, again and again, is the theme of Session 3. The syllabus, the intentions of each element, and associated home practices are summarized in Table 9.1. Mindful movement in MBCT, as in MBSR, is a skilful means to do this. Focusing on sensations in the body is an effective way of "grounding" oneself in the here-and-now and becoming intimate with a new way of knowing: one that is direct rather than mediated by thinking. Mindful movement is also a preparation for practices later in the program that encourage intentionally turning toward the difficult. Later classes will invite turning toward *emotional* difficulties; turning toward physical "edges" in yoga is a good analogy and preparation for this practice. When we first offered MBCT to suicidal people, we learned that the curriculum we had adopted in MBCT for recurrent depression did not meet the need of participants whose urgency to act on their self-destructive thoughts and images is often intense. Let us explain how this realization came about.

Mindful Movement

In MBCT for recurrent depression without suicidal risk (see Segal et al., 2013, p. 181), the class opens with a 5-minute seeing or hearing practice, followed by a 30-minute sitting meditation focusing awareness

TABLE 9.1. Week 3: Summary of Practices

Session theme	Practices and exercises	Skills learned	Insights supported by practices	Home practice
Gathering the scattered mind The mind is often scattered and lost in thought because it is working away in the background to complete unfinished tasks and strive for future goals. Instead, we need to find a way to intentionally "come back" to the here-and-now. The breath and body offer an ever-present focus on which we can reconnect with mindful presence, gather and settle the mind, and ease ourselves from doing into being.	*Yoga stretches* Participants are guided through a series of *yoga stretches* and are encouraged to observe changing bodily sensations during and after each stretch. *Stretch and breath meditation (Audio Track 6ª)* A sequence of standing yoga stretches followed by a shorter sitting meditation in which participants are invited to attend to the constantly changing sensations of the breath, to observe with curiosity wherever the mind wanders, and then to gently return attention to the breath. In the final stages of the practice attention is broadened to the body as a whole.	To become aware of the body in movement, to observe mind wandering during practice, and learn to reconnect with bodily sensations. To attend to the breath, to notice mind wandering, and to become familiar with the habits of the mind. To begin to use the breath as a vehicle to reconnect with present-moment awareness when the mind has wandered.	Bodily sensations are richer and more changeable if observed with full attention. Increasing awareness of habitual patterns of the mind (e.g., the occurrence of striving and related "self-critical" thoughts or difficult bodily sensations). The breath is a route to present-moment awareness.	*Stretch and breath* A sequence of standing yoga stretches followed by a shorter sitting meditation focusing on the breath, completed on days 1, 3, and 5. *Movement (2, 4, 6)* A longer sequence of yoga postures guided by Audio Track 5, completed on days 2, 4, and 6. *Scheduled breathing spaces* Participants practice the 3-minute breathing space (Audio Track 8) on three predetermined occasions each day. *Noticing unpleasant events* Participants are asked to notice events or moments they experience as unpleasant and observe the thoughts, feelings and bodily sensations that arise on these occasions.

146

3-minute breathing space (Audio Track 8)	A 3-minute practice in which participants first become aware of present moment thoughts, feelings and bodily sensations, then shift their attention to the breath, and finally expand their attention to the body as a whole.	To begin to generalize the practice of meditation into everyday life.	It is possible to shift perspective and reconnect with the present moment through the use of the breathing space.

*a*Audio recordings of the guided mindfulness meditation practices used in the MBCT program are available to readers for streaming or downloading at *www.guilford. com/williams6-materials.*

on the breath and then the body, followed later by a sequence of standing stretches (Audio Track 6), and for home practice this alternates with 40 minutes of guided yoga stretches, done lying down. Note that, unlike MBSR, the lying-down yoga is not taught in the session itself in the original MBCT protocol. Why was that change made?

In MBSR, teaching lying-down yoga stretches in class is particularly helpful as many of the participants for whom MBSR was originally developed had been referred by their physicians for significant physical problems. Extended lying-down movement brings them close to the heart of their suffering—to what needs to be "related to differently" for transformation to take place. When MBSR was originally adapted to create MBCT, there was a need to meet the challenge of recurrent depression. In recurrent depression, the center of the suffering is not so much *physical* distress as it is the *ruminative patterns of the mind*. One of the changes made in MBCT was therefore to prioritize sitting practice. The longer sittings are deliberately introduced earlier in MBCT classes and home practice than they were in the original MBSR curriculum: hence MBCT's introduction of a longer sitting with body and breath after a seeing practice at the start of Session 3, and home practice that alternates the lying-down yoga of MBSR with a "stretch and breath" practice (Audio Track 6), rather than a continuing body scan in home practice.

However, we noticed in our early work with suicidal participants that for some, keeping attention focused on the subtle sensations of the body in stillness and on the breath was so significant a challenge that toxic thoughts and feelings became overwhelming. Sometimes, it was simply impossible for them to remain in contact with the often minimal body sensations in the body scan and long sittings. The experience of one participant, Rowena, in one of our early classes of MBCT for people at risk of suicide, is a good example of what prompted us to change what we did in Session 3, to come back to MBSR's emphasis on teaching lying-down yoga stretches—though retaining the alternating home practice. Let us describe her experience

Rowena's Story

Rowena was an "unplanned" baby, and her parents made this clear to her. If she did anything wrong as a small child, or got into an argument with them as she was growing up, they would say that they hadn't wanted her anyway—that she was a mistake. She grew up feeling she had no place in the world. She had many problems early in life and had been a rebellious child, but her first bout of depression was at age 12, when a close friend moved away. For a time, she felt life was simply not worth living—her friend's departure seemed to confirm her sense of being a complete outsider, unloved and unwanted. By the time she came to the classes, Rowena was in her late 20s, and she had experienced a number of episodes of serious depression, of which suicidal thoughts and impulses had become a regular feature. Something would go wrong (particularly anything that might signal rejection by someone she cared about), and she would plunge swiftly into hopelessness, self-hatred, and despair. She had attempted suicide on two occasions, the most recent being a few months before she came to class. She said she wanted desperately to get out of this cycle, but was terrified that it would all start up again and this time it would be the end. In the first 3 weeks, Rowena really struggled with the body scan and sitting meditations (her mind was constantly pulled away and her moods became dangerously worse) but her reaction to the mindful movement practices was dramatically different. Here at last she could see a glimmer of hope:

> "This yoga stuff was a revelation to me. I had such a hard time with the body scan, my mind was off and wouldn't come back. But with the stretches, for the first time, I could more or less keep my attention on what I was doing. I could really feel my body, because of the movement and the stretching. There were really strong sensations, and I felt I was right there with them. I had two horrible days in the middle of the week, and the old stuff started up—'it was all my fault,' 'Things would never change,' and on and on. So I did the yoga practice twice every day, and bits of it at other times when I could, and I found I could still pay attention, and not get blown away by my feelings. They didn't go, but they were more in the background, sort of, I didn't get so tangled up in them."

On the basis of reports like this, we decided to alter the structure of Session 3. Participants encountered mindful movement twice. First, we restored the 40 minutes of stretches lying down that remains an integral part of the MBSR curriculum (Kabat-Zinn, 2013), and we also retained the standing stretches (followed by sitting with breath and body) that had become part of MBCT. Our sense was that, for people like Rowena, experiencing a range of different movement practices during the class itself (as well as for home practice) might offer a more fluent access to mindful awareness even when things were tough. Just as she described, the relatively powerful sensations of the body moving might hold the attention when the slight movement of the breath might not—a sort of mindfully chosen, conscious distraction in the midst of the storm, an act of kindness and nurturance at times when it is most needed.

The instructions for both mindful movement practices invite participants to experience movement in a particular way.

"This is a mindful movement practice and, just like the body scan, the intention is not to try to achieve any particular goal, but rather to become minutely aware of changing patterns of sensation as the body moves, stretches, and returns to stillness. This is not an exercise class, we're not here to become fitter or stronger or more flexible—in fact, we're not striving to change things at all, but rather to tune into how things are, moment by moment. It's important to be sensitive to your body's limitations—to respect them rather than feeling you have to push beyond them. All you need do is open your awareness to whatever sensations are present, exploring your body, just as it is. And exploring your 'edges,' your limits, just as they are today. Neither backing off as soon as you sense discomfort or tiredness, nor driving yourself beyond your body's boundaries. Simply attending to your experience in each moment, whatever it may be."

Mindful Movement as a Model for and Embodiment of "Moving in Close" to Pain and Discomfort

The increased focus on mindful movement (Audio Track 5) offered early opportunities to explore physically as well as emotionally the felt sense of turning toward difficulty, or "working at our edge." The body provides an important place to experience how, when challenge arises, "enough is enough" for now. This "edge" might be experienced as hardness or solidity, tightness, painful sensations of sharpness or heat, or a bodily realization of limit as there is no possibility to move forward in this moment. Participants are encouraged to discover how this "edge" can manifest both in the body and also in the mind, for example, when, as the body moves into a particular posture, thoughts arise such as "I can't do this!", "My body wouldn't ever be able to do that movement/stretch!", "This is too much," or simply "No!"

As we have seen, mindful movement can provide a chance to experience intense sensations and emotional responses. Here the group are asked explicitly to explore the possibility of turning toward intense experiences, created intentionally, by engaging in mindful stretching. As Vidyamala Burch (2008) points out in her work on living with physical pain, the nature of the experience of being "at an edge" can be discovered so that many feel the difference between *hard* edges where it is not wise to push further and in contrast the *soft* edges where, if you pause, gently and kindly play with or ease toward these edges, there can be surprising amounts of movement, flexibility and openness. The paradox of experiencing how easing into intense solidity can radically shift *edges* or *limits* offers important learning. The physicality of this learning can offer a new doorway to approaching the "edges" of powerful thoughts and emotions. The transferability of this learning is sometimes immediately clear to people in classes: this practice is a microcosm of experience in life. Habitual reactive patterns of body and mind may be seen in mindful movement as the tendency to push against or alternatively retreat from edges in everyday experience and there can be the recognition: "Ah . . . here I am doing what I do!"

Breathing Space

During Session 3, as in the original MBCT, the 3-minute breathing space (Audio Track 8) is introduced (see the sidebar on p. 152). It retains the aims and intentions that give it a central place in MBCT. It is a means of bringing meditation practice into everyday life, a moment to pause in the flow of things and step out of automatic pilot, and then to take three steps: for participants to change *how* they relate to their experience (acknowledging and being curious in Step 1—What is here for me now? Thoughts? Emotions? Sensations?), to change *what* they focus on (gathering the focus of attention to the breath in the lower abdomen—Step 2), then to change the *view* they take of experience (expanding the focus of attention to include *all* experience—Step 3) before reentering the flow of daily living.

As in MBCT, in the inquiry we emphasize that this is not so much about distraction, relaxation, or "fixing," but about stepping out of automatic pilot and seeing clearly what is present in this moment, anchored by the breath. It encourages awareness of the activity of mind and body in everyday life, facilitates approaching the next moment in a new way, from a wider perspective, and thereby becomes a first step to choosing how best to respond to crises, on the basis of clear seeing rather than old habits of thought.

In teaching the breathing space in class we saw again and again the *need for precision in describing the three steps, for example, actually saying* "Step 1 . . . ; Step 2 . . . ; Step 3 . . ." as part of the guidance to make its structure clear. *It also became very clear how important it was to keep it short and straightforward,* simply instructing participants on what to attend to, without elaboration.

THE THREE STEPS OF THE BREATHING SPACE

The three distinct steps of the breathing space assist participants to see clearly and then to shift in three aspects: the *how*, the *what*, and the *view* of moment-to-moment experience.

In acknowledging what's on the mind and in the body without attempting to change it (Step 1) there is an immediate and natural shift from the more automatic reaction of aversion to a sense of curiosity and interest (the *"how"* has changed).

In coming to the breath (Step 2) there is a gathering and focusing that brings the newly developing skills of calm grounding to the situation through changing the content of the mind (the *"what"* has changed).

In the wider awareness of the body (Step 3) the preparation to return to the world is done through widening the focus of awareness so the next moment is more likely to be viewed not through the contracted mind of striving and aversion, but the more open presence of allowing (the *"view"* has changed).

See Teasdale et al. (2014, p. 100).

The breathing space has become the most important practice in MBCT. During the course, the breathing space develops to become the spine of the program, the means by which what is being learned in formal practices are incorporated into everyday life. Here is a summary of its use as home practice:

- Session 3: Routine breathing spaces (three times daily from this point in the program).
- Session 4: Additional breathing spaces (same format as routine breathing spaces, but used when experiencing distress or discomfort).
- Session 5: Expanded breathing space (additional instructions to aid observation of present-moment experience, to facilitate focused attention to the breath, and to allow all experience to be present including difficulty or discomfort).
- Session 6: Breathing space as a prelude to attending to thoughts as mental events.
- Session 7: Breathing space as a prelude to taking wise action in the presence of difficulty and emotional pain, and, for our participants, the presence of despair and the urge to escape through suicide or self-harm.

So, when setting up the breathing space for home practice in class, it is important to ensure time for participants to plan when they will incorporate it into their day. We will not discuss the breathing space further. For more on its use in MBCT, see Segal et al. (2013, Ch. 18) and Teasdale et al. (2014, Ch. 7).

Unpleasant Experiences Diary

This exercise is the first in the MBCT curriculum that explicitly and intentionally introduces exploration of difficult experiences. It is introduced toward the end of Session 3, and completed daily as home practice during the week. Often there may be some reluctance and hesitation around this invitation to focus on experiences of difficulty. Nonetheless, as we have seen, participants vulnerable to suicidal depression may in fact have already been exploring difficulty throughout the course. It is not uncommon for them to predict that this will be an easier task than the pleasant experiences diary, as awareness of the unpleasant is familiar to them, and so it sometimes proved.

Just as with the pleasant experiences diary, it will be important in reviewing this home practice during Session 4 to attend closely to the different elements of unpleasantness: thoughts, feelings, body sensations, and impulses. It is especially important to tune in to how the body feels at such times, as later in the program the body is increasingly used as the place to return to in order to explore difficult experiences.

Concluding Remarks

In Session 3, highly vulnerable participants discover a different form of mindfulness: awareness of the body in motion rather than in stillness. For some, the focus on mindful movement offers moments of respite in the midst of turmoil; the power of the sensations can encourage sustained attention in a way that stillness and the subtlety of the breath may not. Again, we focus on carrying mindfulness into everyday life, both through the breathing space and through the home practice focusing on everyday unpleasant experiences. Here is a gentle move toward the heart of Session 4: turning toward depression itself.

CHAPTER 10

Session 4: Recognizing Aversion

Session 4

The curriculum of Session 4 continues the theme of seeing clearly how difficult mind states have different yet interacting elements: thoughts, feelings, physical sensations, and behaviors, and aims to deepen this understanding by exploring the way in which the mind reacts to aversion. The syllabus, the intentions of each element, and associated home practices are summarized in Table 10.1.

First, there is a long sitting meditation (Kabat-Zinn, 2013, Ch. 4, pp. 73–74; Teasdale et al., 2014) in which participants are invited to focus first on the breath, then on the body as a whole (as they have practiced before); but then to move on to mindfulness of sounds, then to thought and feelings (Audio Track 11). This is the first time that people have intentionally made an extended space to notice the arising and passing away of thoughts and feelings in formal practice.

Participants sometimes describe the moment when they are invited to bring thoughts center-stage in the sitting meditation as the exact moment when, paradoxically, thoughts dissolve in awareness. All these thoughts that have been calling for attention suddenly vanish—for a few moments at least. Thoughts have felt like a constant violent knocking on the door until this point but, once the door has been opened wide, not only does the knocking stop but the thoughts that have been calling for attention have run away and hidden! Just

TABLE 10.1. Week 4: Summary of Practices

Session theme	Practices and exercises	Skills learned	Insights supported by practices	Home practice
Recognizing aversion Aim: To begin the experiential investigation of *aversion*—the mind's habitual reaction to unpleasant. To explore how the skill of "coming back" needs to be complemented by seeing more clearly what "takes us away" into doing, rumination, mind wandering and worry feelings and sensations, driven by the need not to have these experiences, which is at the root of emotional suffering. Mindfulness offers a way of staying present by giving another way to view things: it helps us take a wider perspective and relate differently to experience.	*Seeing meditation/hearing meditation* A short meditation practice in which participants focus attention on either sights or sounds, returning attention gently to these sensations whenever the mind wanders. *Sitting meditation* A sitting meditation (Audio Track 11) in which the focus is initially on the *breath*, moving then to the *body as a whole*. Participants are encouraged to explore intense sensations with an attitude of openness and curiosity, as an alternative to changing position to alleviate discomforts. Attention then moves to *sounds*, and to *thoughts/feelings*, and finally to whatever is salient in awareness from moment to moment (*"choiceless awareness"*).	To include sights or sounds as the object of awareness. To practice shifting out of automatic pilot and tuning in to different aspects of moment-to-moment experience. To begin to explore the possibility of staying with difficult sensations, seeing our own "aversion signatures" and adopting an attitude of curiosity, openness, and acceptance.	It is possible to use awareness of sights and sounds to step out of automatic pilot and reconnect with the present moment. Attention to sights or sounds can be particularly "grounding." When one chooses to stay with difficult sensations rather than trying to eradicate them, it is possible to notice their qualities in more detail. Sometimes difficult sensations spontaneously change.	*Sitting meditation* A sitting meditation (Audio Track 11[a]) in which the object of attention shifts from breath, to body, to sounds, to thoughts, and finally to choiceless awareness. *Breathing spaces* Participants are encouraged to take 3-minute breathing spaces (Audio Track 8) not only on three scheduled occasions but also at times when they notice distress or emotional pressure mounting.

156

Automatic Thoughts Questionnaire

Participants read through the questionnaire to explore the most common dysfunctional and negative thoughts that occur in depression. They also review the DSM symptoms of major depression.

To recognize negative and dysfunctional thoughts. To reflect on these symptoms from a metacognitive perspective.

The negative thoughts and experiences that accompany depression are recognized symptoms, not signs of personal weakness or unique to the individual.

Mindful walking

Participants are instructed in the practice of *walking meditation* (Audio Track 7), attending to the sensations arising from the movement and placement of the feet and legs. Pace is usually slow. Attention is redirected to the body when the mind wanders.

To become aware of the body in movement, and learn to reconnect with bodily sensations when the mind wanders.

[a]Audio recordings of the guided mindfulness meditation practices used in the MBCT program are available to readers for streaming or downloading at *www.guilford.com/williams6-materials*.

as suddenly, thoughts and images can appear again with great force, accompanied by feelings that seem to validate them. So, for example, the *thought* "I can't bear this anymore" comes along with a *feeling* of despair that seems to authenticate the thought and make it impossible to see as a mental event—it seems to be telling the truth and to demand immediate action.

Sharon Salzberg uses the metaphor of a teaspoon of salt in a small glass of water compared to the same amount in a lake to describe this phenomenon. A teaspoon of salt would make a glass of water difficult to drink, but the same teaspoonful dropped in a freshwater lake would make no difference to the taste. In the same way, space created around intense experiences can create a felt sense of diluting their intensity.

> Our true work is to create a container so immense that any amount of salt, even a truckload, can come into it without affecting our capacity to receive it. No situation, even an extreme one, then can mandate a particular reaction. (Salzberg, 1995, p. 43)

For some in MBCT classes the introduction of this focus on unpleasant experiences ends a honeymoon period of mindfulness as a way to just be with the pleasantness of life and feel more relaxed and connected to daily experiences. As would be expected, some discomfort, resistance, and avoidance can arise. This was even more so in the classes for suicidal depression. By now the group have become a little more familiar with mindfully noticing experiences, beginning to acknowledge and recognize the interconnections between thought, body sensations, emotions, and behaviors, even when things challenge them. But getting rid of unpleasant mind and body states seems more urgent for these participants—and the reaction to them can be extreme. We saw this in the exercise of looking at automatic thoughts.

Automatic Thoughts Questionnaire

The Automatic Thoughts Questionnaire (ATQ; Hollon & Kendall, 1980) lists cognitions frequently reported by people suffering from depression (see Table 10.2). In Session 4, we used a slightly modified version of this questionnaire as a jumping-off point for an exercise exploring the relationship between thinking and depression.

TABLE 10.2. The Voice of Depression Speaking: The Automatic Thoughts Questionnaire (ATQ)

Listed below are a variety of thoughts that pop into people's heads. Please read the list, and notice what happens as you do so. Do you recognize any of them? Which thoughts feel most familiar to you? When you feel very low, how often do thoughts like these occur? And how far do you believe them? How convincing do they seem? And what about when you are feeling well? How often do the thoughts occur then? And how far do you believe them? How convincing do they feel?

1. I feel like I'm up against the world.
2. I'm no good.
3. Why can't I ever succeed?
4. No one understands me.
5. I've let people down.
6. I don't think I can go on.
7. I wish I were a better person.
8. I'm so weak.
9. My life's not going the way I want it to.
10. I'm so disappointed in myself.
11. Nothing feels good anymore.
12. I can't stand this anymore.
13. I can't get started.
14. What's wrong with me?
15. I wish I were somewhere else.
16. I can't get things together.
17. I hate myself.
18. I'm worthless.
19. I wish I could just disappear.
20. What's the matter with me?
21. I'm a loser.
22. My life is mess.
23. I'm a failure.
24. I'll never make it.
25. I feel so helpless.
26. Something has to change.
27. There must be something wrong with me.
28. My future is bleak.
29. It's just not worth it.
30. I can't finish anything.

When we feel low, thoughts like these often feel like "the truth" about us. But in fact they are symptoms of depression—just as a high temperature is a symptom of flu. Becoming aware, through mindfulness, that they are just "the voice of depression speaking" allows us to step back from them and begin to choose whether to take them seriously or not. Perhaps, in fact, we can learn simply to notice them, acknowledge their presence, and let them go.

Note. From Hollon and Kendall (1980). Reprinted with permission from the authors and Springer Science + Business Media.

This part of the class can offer a powerful reminder of the close and rapid connections between thought and mood, body, and behavior for anyone with a history of depression. Reading the list of standard depressive thoughts on a printed piece of paper may have little effect on some who feel no connection to them, finding it hard to imagine ever believing these thoughts from their current state of being well. For others, however, it may trigger profound mood shifts. The printed sheet provides for them a reconnection to the threat, now present in the room, of the toxic thoughts so familiar to them from episodes of depression.

Christine, once she had read the list, curled up into a ball with her feet drawn up onto the chair. This reaction had happened quickly and automatically, with no sense of her having chosen to do so. This, and other physical reactions present in the room, were noted by the teacher. The sense of the group's retreat into other times and places of avoidance and present-moment habitual patterns of thinking and feeling was often palpable. Here it was: they had retreated from this perceived threat in an instant.

It is important to acknowledge that exploring such depressed thinking can evoke powerful emotions; reading and reflecting on the ATQ in effect constitutes a sort of mood induction (and recall that mood induction is associated for the most vulnerable participants with a "closing down" of options). There is a sense of deep, and often painful, engagement—shown sometimes in increased energy and agitation, sometimes by a collapse in energy—reflecting the seemingly overwhelming power of "the voice of depression speaking." Notice that this can happen even when participants are well, in the relative safety of a class, with a trusted teacher, and with an explicit message that even these painful thoughts are no more than aspects of a particular human mind state which can perhaps (with practice) be responded to with recognition, acknowledgment, and kindness. Teachers too feel this quality of despair and mental anguish. Their intention is to relieve suffering, not to cause people pain. It may feel as if inviting participants to experience difficult and distressing thoughts and feelings stands in direct opposition to this healing intention. The saving grace is the confidence, deriving from theory and deepened through experience, that only by making contact with painful thoughts and feelings can participants see them clearly, understand them fully, and develop new, transformative responses to them. This is essential to fulfilling the program's central intention: helping people to stay well.

In our work with people at risk of suicide, at these challenging moments, our trust in and clear understanding of the intention of this work were central. Here was an opportunity to practice ourselves, feeling the impact here-and-now, remaining open and curious, grounded, anchored in the physicality of our feet on the floor, our bodies on our seats, and the breath moving in the body. Supporting ourselves with practice at these moments was crucial to holding suffering, fear, and despair—in others and in ourselves. Our embodiment of this gentle but confident holding of distress offered potential for significant learning: it is safe to feel and be with even this level of painful emotion.

Thus powerfully emotive moments are both the most challenging but also offer some of the greatest opportunities to connect learning *about* mindfulness to being mindful of *direct experience* for this group. Here is a chance to invite the group to decenter and see this process *in vivo*. As we say in the class, these thoughts arise for people with depression just as a high temperature arises with flu. So, the relevance of this learning could come into clear focus. "This is why this approach might help me."

We take a breathing space in class after the ATQ exercise to deepen the possibility of learning from it. The choice to ground, become present with the immediacy of experiences in the body, here and now, gives a chance to use the breathing space in action: not to fix the bad feelings, but to acknowledge them, ground oneself, then expand the sense of space around the feelings (allowing the participants to "reenter" the class with an expanded rather than a contracted view).

James said at the end of the ATQ exercise and breathing space:

"Wow, that was powerful! I think I usually just get lost inside it when I feel that bad. I've never really noticed my experience in those moments like that. It brought to mind a time when I was on a beach in springtime when it was really foggy. I thought the fog must be covering the whole area but when I stepped outside I could see how small the area really was."

Mindful Walking

Mindful walking (Audio Track 7) was in the original MBCT proto-col as an optional additional home practice but, like the lying-down stretches, was not taught in the class. We decided it was too impor-tant to leave out (and spoken guidance for walking meditation is now provided as part of the MBCT Workbook downloads: see Teasdale, Williams, & Segal, 2014). We scheduled a mindful walking practice following the ATQ and the breathing space. The aim was to allow par-ticipants to further extend their sense of being able to shift attentional focus and anchor themselves in body sensations. Focusing on the body in movement helps participants to make a shift from the habitual "tightening and closing" that the body is inclined to do in its reaction to the threat of these thoughts. This in turn offered a clear invitation to let go of the thoughts the ATQ had triggered, not by suppressing them, but rather by intentionally refocusing attention elsewhere: to the body in the present moment. The process of letting go, cognitively and physically, could be seen clearly by all of us.

Mindful walking involves walking at a slower pace than normal, with the attention narrowly focused on the contact between the soles of the feet and the floor. This encourages close and detailed observa-tion of the sensations of walking. It is followed by inquiry into partici-pants' experiences:

> TEACHER: Would anyone be willing to share their experience of that practice?
>
> ROZ: I never realized walking was so difficult! I kept thinking I was going to fall over. I would never normally walk that slowly.
>
> TEACHER: Yes, indeed. No wonder it took such a time to learn how to do it when we were small! It's a really complex process, isn't it? Did anyone notice anything else?
>
> PHIL: I was really interested to notice how much is involved—I was focusing on my feet, but I could feel all sorts of muscles constantly moving, and my breathing too in the background.
>
> TEACHER: It sounds like you haven't noticed that before?
>
> PHIL: No, I don't think so. Normally I'm not paying attention, I'm

thinking about where I have to get to, or something that just happened, or whatever.

TEACHER: The mind is elsewhere, and you're walking on automatic pilot. Just as we discovered with the raisin, back in the first class. It's a really interesting practice, because of course we all do lots of walking in everyday life. With practice, we can learn to bring the same kind of careful attention to any walking, making mindful awareness part of everyday life. At any moment, you can choose to bring attention to the soles of the feet, literally to "ground" yourself.

Concluding Remarks

By the end of Session 4, participants are much more familiar with the territory into which we are choosing to venture together. They have come half-way in the 8-week program, exploring little by little a new way to hold the full range of experience with spacious, kindly care. This is gradually opening up the possibility of allowing them both to see clearly and to choose skillfully how best to respond, even to what is difficult. The observation of how things are in this moment is the chosen focus, the stepping back or decentering to hold it all just as it is; the detail of the experience is secondary.

Participants can see more clearly that pain and risk are a part of their experience. Past memories may arise and habitual patterns can reestablish themselves at any moment. These experiences are not simply something that people are bound to encounter as they learn mindfulness meditation, but something that we explicitly invite people to contact. Learning to relate in a new way to painful material is essential if they are to remain well. Baer's (2003) meta-analysis pointed to *exposure* as one of the factors of change in mindfulness, a willingness to turn toward what might ordinarily be avoided or suppressed in order to experience it, investigate it, and see it clearly. In the continual unfolding, the impermanence of experience is understood, not simply as pleasant or unpleasant, not fixed in time or nature, but constantly evolving.

The human tendency to avoid difficult experience means inevitably that very little may be known about its true nature in the present moment. Mindfulness practice offers many opportunities to explore, define, and understand the nature of experiences that participants find particularly challenging. They learn to see clearly the universal qualities of such difficult experiences and to witness the subtleties of how these experiences can be refracted within the mind/body through perception, interpretations, and reactivity.

Mindfulness practice helps participants to observe processes that are either ancient and hard-wired or overlearned and habitual as they arise and influence our internal experience and behavior. Through practice, they feel their power and persuasiveness and notice reactions to them: "This is dangerous." For our participants, the strength of emotions may be so great it feels as though it absolutely *must* be true and worth believing. "What do you mean, notice *this*? I can't focus on the present moment if things stay like *this*!" They learn how to work with automatic, "kneejerk" reactions, how to stay steady in their presence, to investigate, and so to become familiar with them. From this kindly, decentered perspective, people begin to perceive choices, the possibility of new, mindful responses. Sessions 1–4 have laid the foundations, teaching people how they might ground themselves in the face of overwhelming emotions. It is time to encourage participants to go further—to go beyond *noticing* their own aversion, to deliberately allowing it, turning toward it, and exploring it. In this work, kind and steady attending to the body will be their greatest ally.

CHAPTER 11

Session 5:
Allowing/Letting Be

The repeated mindfulness meditation practice of Sessions 1–4 aims to establish a foundation of relatively settled awareness, as well as the capacity to notice and release passing thoughts and feelings, and to let go of other diversions from the intended point of focus. This increase in a clearer, more direct awareness can feel both appropriate and welcome to many participants in a mindfulness course, and can have the effect of increasing a sense of being alive. From eating mindfully, to seeing what is around them when walking from one room to another at work or at home, people often report feeling increasing awareness of the *pleasant* in their lives in its many shapes and forms. Realization that these aspects of life are already present and available—it is just a matter of turning toward and seeing them—is frequently described as both liberating and exciting. Tuning in to and making time and space to explore pleasant experiences offers us a different, broader view of our lives. For some comes a realization: perhaps all that needs to change is the way we view things; much is already perfect just the way it is. The first four sessions can be a turning point for many. At the same time, understanding of the nature of depressed and suicidal thinking and the ability to decenter from it are growing.

But this is not always the case. As we have already seen, the first few sessions are when many of participants who are at risk of suicide would tend to leave. They find even the idea of mindfulness difficult and the actual practice intolerable. Now, with the additional preparation that they are receiving in the preclass interview, those who are most at risk stay, and are still there at the end of Session 4. At this point, there is a further transition, and it is a shift that almost all participants in any mindfulness program find challenging: the invitation to turn toward or make more space for experiences that are *un*pleasant or difficult. This step has to be taken, however. The training in conscious attentional deployment experienced in Sessions 1–4 builds the "base camp" from which to venture out, intentionally, toward the difficult in Sessions 5–8: investigating its resonances in the body (Session 5), in thought (Session 6), and in wise action and self-nurture (Session 7).

Doubts and Challenges in Turning toward the Difficult

Our participants were people for whom there was an ongoing and significant risk of triggering depressive feelings and suicidal impulses. As teachers, this was often at the forefront in our discussions and supervisions, especially around the Session 5 transition, when MBCT offers an intentional invitation to turn toward difficult experience. Would this not create unnecessary risk for these participants? Would the methods and practices involved justify the risks? It was crucial for us to understand the deep competencies involved in skilled mindfulness teaching (see Chapter 16) and how these specifically related to people with suicidal depression. We trusted mindfulness to be appropriate for people with a history of recurrent depression (through our own research evidence, our experiences of mindfulness, our practice, and our teaching experiences), and we knew that there were reasons for cautious optimism that it would also be valuable to those whose depression included suicidal thinking, but subjectively we felt we needed more understanding and experience to extend the practice to these highly vulnerable participants.

The tendency for this client group to live predominantly in their conceptual, *driven-doing* mode of mind and to return there when threat arises has been described in Part I (see Chapters 2 and 4). Thinking is a particularly pernicious mode for this client group where memories, powerful self-attacking images, thoughts of hopelessness and being trapped, feelings of overwhelming helplessness, and despair feature strongly. As we have seen, the evolved human mind sees and feels the *inner* reality created by thoughts in just the same way as the evolutionarily ancient mind reacted to actual *external* reality—triggering fear and avoidant helplessness and thus reducing the possibility of creative and effective response strategies. The people attending our classes had experienced depression repeatedly, and with it despair, entrapment, and suicidal impulses.

Recognizing the particular difficulties our vulnerable participants might experience with this shift of emphasis encouraged us to make specific changes to Session 5. First, we offered an opportunity to reflect on the mental pain of despair, those crisis moments when life no longer seems worth living and suicide may appear the most desirable option. Second, we explored patterns of behavior that are intended to provide relief but may unwittingly keep mental and emotional pain in place.

> "Turning toward the difficult" is a tender "making space to move closer." But how? It helps to know that all such experiences are multifaceted when seen in close detail—amalgams of thoughts, body sensations, emotions, and behaviors or urges. Seeing and feeling more clearly in this way brings new perspectives, so even when nothing seems to change, something profound happens— there may be a glimpse that it can be worked with, and that's enough for now.

Session 5

The syllabus, the intentions of each element, and associated home practices are summarized in Table 11.1.

In accordance with the original MBCT program that was our model (Segal et al., 2002), Session 5 opened with a sitting meditation, focusing awareness on the breath and then the body (Audio Track 12). During this practice, participants were invited to turn toward a difficulty already present in body or mind, and to explore how it expressed itself in the body, in particular noticing signs of aversion (tightening, bracing, pulling away). This practice offers participants an opportunity to relate to difficulty in a new way, allowing it to be present and, with a sense of compassion, gently exploring its physical expression while "breathing into" bodily aversion and allowing it to release and soften as

TABLE 11.1. Week 5: Summary of Practices

Session theme	Practices and exercises	Skills learned	Insights supported by practices	Home practice
Allowing/ letting be	*Sitting meditation*	To begin to explore the possibility of staying with and accepting difficult thoughts, images, memories, emotions, and body sensations.	Difficult experiences may have bodily manifestations that can be observed.	*Working with difficulty meditation*
Aim: To begin to develop a radically different relationship to experience in which all experiences are allowed and accepted.	A meditation in which participants bring attention first to the breath, then to wider awareness of sensations in the body as a whole. Participants are invited to notice if the mind returns repeatedly to certain themes to bring a curiosity and openness to these. Participants are encouraged to deliberately bring a difficulty to mind and notice how it is expressed in the body, to become aware of tensions or other bodily sensations associated with difficulty and to use the breath as a vehicle to stay with these experiences in an open way, "breathing into and out from" regions where the difficulties are manifesting themselves not to change the sensations but rather to help soften the relationship to them.	To observe how difficulties manifest themselves in the body. To observe our usual tendency to attempt to suppress or avoid unpleasant experiences or to try to fix difficulties and to practice an alternative approach.	By staying with difficulties rather than attempting to avoid them or change them, change sometimes occurs spontaneously.	A guided meditation (Audio Track 12[a]) following the format of the sitting meditation practiced in the class. *Sitting in stillness* An unguided 30–40 minute sitting meditation in which patients guide their own practice. *Breathing spaces* Participants continue to practice both scheduled breathing spaces (Audio Track 8) and spontaneous breathing spaces at times of stress or difficulty, with added instructions for each step of the breathing space and specific focus in Step 3 on how difficulties are manifest in the body (Audio Track 9).

[a]Audio recordings of the guided mindfulness meditation practices used in the MBCT program are available to readers for streaming or downloading at *www.guilford. com/williams6-materials*.

168

best they can. If no difficulty is present, they may choose deliberately to introduce one into their awareness (e.g., a worry, irritation, or concern) and follow the same process with this. A downloadable track for this "Working with Difficulty Meditation" (Audio Track 12) is included in *The Mindful Way Workbook* (Teasdale et al., 2014).

"Sitting with the difficult" is part of a broader Session 5 focus on painful experiences and different—more or less helpful—ways of responding to them. We wished to extend the curriculum to ensure that we included a number of elements that would get close to the heart of what maintains the suffering of the suicidal person—the rumination and avoidance and associated collapse of problem solving.

Recognizing Mental Pain

For people at risk of suicide, the depressed thinking we had investigated in Session 4 was not the whole story. Many also experience moments of vast emotional turmoil, crisis points where the option of suicide is intensely present. This was why the assessment process had included preparing a crisis card (see pp. 88–89). We knew that these moments of crisis might be triggered with great speed by apparently trivial events or shifts in mood or body state, resulting in a collapse of problem-solving capacity, perceived loss of a viable future, and perhaps powerful images of previous suicidal plans or impulses, with the sense of unfinished business pulling them to take action ("flashforward"). The resulting "tunnel vision" might lead to a sense that there was only one possible way forward: suicide. We realized that it was necessary to address this issue openly, as we had done with individual participants in our preclass interviews:

> "Last week, we reflected on the kind of thinking that emerges when depression arises, and how compelling and true these thoughts seem even though in fact, as we discovered, they are the reflection of a particular mood state, the voice of depression speaking. There are some moments that are particularly hard to bear—those moments when pain is intense, when toxic thoughts and frightening images and memories crowd in, and when it seems as if there is no way out and nothing will ever change for the better. Do these sound familiar to you?

"Today we will look more closely at these very difficult times. Might it be possible to hold even these darkest moments in awareness, to turn toward them just as you turned toward difficulty in our sitting practice today, to hold steady in their presence and to be gentle and compassionate even to this? Two things can make this especially difficult—the power of the thoughts and feelings, and the reactions that spring from this power, reactions that we hope against hope will help, but that may in fact unintentionally have just the opposite effect. Let us explore these together."

Pain and Suffering

We adapted the Buddha's parable of the two arrows (Chapter 3, pp. 33–34), elaborating it into an image of *three* arrows, all striking the same point and representing factors likely to deepen the pain of despair. These can be drawn on the whiteboard (see Figure 11.1), and are:

- Sheer intensity of feeling, so that (like intense physical pain) it becomes all-consuming.
- Meanings attached to the pain (e.g., "This is my fault," "No one can help me," "This will never end").

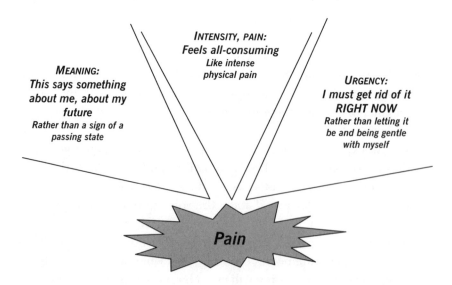

FIGURE 11.1. The arrows of mental pain (option for drawing on the board).

- A sense of urgency to do something–anything–to relieve the pain, right now.

This image can be used to open an exploration of how the people in the class might typically react to the experience of pain, and what the intentions and actual outcomes of those reactions might be.

Finding Alternatives to Self-Defeating Reactions

"When things are at their worst, I don't know where to turn. It feels as if there is a knife twisting in my guts. I'm being bombarded by all these voices in my head, beating me up, telling me I'll never amount to anything, people would be better off without me, it's never going to get better, it's always going to be like this. All the other times when this has happened come back. And such a turmoil of feelings–not just depression, that's the least of it–guilt because I shouldn't be putting myself through this again, terrible shame, absolute rage that it won't leave me alone and no one seems able to help. I would do anything to get rid of it all. Anything. Killing myself would be a relief. I honestly feel that sometimes. . . ." (Leyla)

In the presence of such pain, who would not feel a desperate urge to blot the torment out, to suppress the pain, or numb it, or strive to analyze it out of existence? Out of this urgent need arise patterns of behavior that *feel as if* they will help and indeed may do so, at least in the short term. But in the long run they may feed into future pain and create barriers to real transformation. To clarify this process, we introduced a new interactive exercise, the "vicious flower," detailed below. Its intention is to help participants to refine their awareness of potentially unhelpful reactions to pain, and to develop their confidence to be steady in the presence of powerful thoughts and feelings, and bring curiosity and compassion to them rather than unwittingly adding extra suffering. The teacher's embodiment of steady kindness and confidence, his or her willingness to approach and explore, are foundational in communicating without words that approaching this pain is safe, wise, and helpful–and doesn't have to happen all at once– a toe in the water is fine. This is like practicing mindful movement, learning when to move up close and when to back off a little.

The "Vicious Flower"

The "vicious flower" illustrates how old strategies for dealing with distress do not always have their intended outcome, and is so called because it is made up of vicious circles and the final result looks rather like a flower (see Figure 11.2). This visual (and thus memorable) formulation is drawn from cognitive therapy, where it was first used in relation to health anxiety, and has since been applied to depression and to anxiety disorders in a more general sense.

STAGE 1: IDENTIFYING REACTIONS TO PAIN

The teacher invites participants to call to mind times when they have experienced pain and distress.

> TEACHER: Let us begin with a breathing space. (*Leads breathing space.*) Now, as you sit, aware of breath and body, taking a moment to call to mind times when you experience pain—it

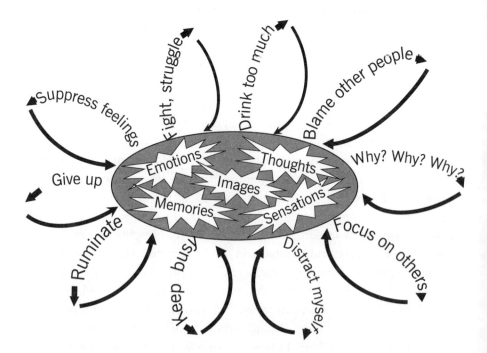

FIGURE 11.2. The "vicious flower": Reactions that keep people stuck in distress.

could be painful thoughts, or images, or memories. (*pause*) Or perhaps painful emotions. (*pause*) Or body sensations. (*pause*) And calling to mind how, at those times, you normally react. What do you do to relieve the pain, to control or manage it? (*pause*) When you're ready, opening your eyes. (*Moves to the whiteboard, draws a circle, and writes "pain" in it.*) So would anyone be willing to give an example of how you normally react when pain is present?

LEYLA: I try to distract myself, stop myself thinking about it.

TEACHER: (*Draws an arrow outward from circle and writes.*) "Distract myself." Thank you. Another example perhaps?

ROZ: I go the other way—I get caught up in trying to find a way out.

TEACHER: (*Draws an outward arrow and writes.*) "Caught up in finding a way out." Thank you. Do you mean going over and over possible solutions?

ROZ: Yes, over and over.

TEACHER: Another example?

The teacher continues to collect examples from the group and write them on the board encircling "pain" until there is a good range, as shown in Figure 11.2, where the arrows radiating out from the center all represent attempts to escape from or resolve the pain. This discussion is often lively, with a strong (and sometimes humorous) sense of recognizing shared strategies.

STAGE 2: EXPLORING THE INTENTION OF REACTIONS

The teacher then investigates the intentions behind these various reactions:

TEACHER: Okay, thanks for all those examples. So can I ask you why you choose these particular ways of coping?

ROZ: Well, how else am I ever going to get myself out of this hole? There must be a solution somewhere.

PHIL: That's why I go over and over it in my head. Why has this happened again, what'll I do if it goes on? I really want to understand what's going on, and maybe this time I'll make sense of it all.

ROZ: Yes, exactly. (*nods from other participants*)

TEACHER: Thanks. (*to Leyla*) Now, you told us you try to distract yourself, and it looked like quite a few people recognized that one. What would be your reason for doing that? What might happen if you didn't?

LEYLA: I'm afraid if I didn't I'd go on feeling worse and worse, and in the end I'd go crazy.

ADAM: With me, it's that in the end I just wouldn't be able to stand it anymore, it would be too much for me, and I'd end up killing myself. And I can't do that, because of my children.

TEACHER: (*gently*) So when you do all these things, you're trying to look after yourselves, to care for yourselves in the best way you can think of. Is that what's happening?

STAGE 3: EXPLORING SHORT- AND LONG-TERM OUTCOMES

People's strategies are their best attempts to care for themselves in moments of crisis, to deal with the turmoil of thoughts and feelings they are experiencing. So the intention is both understandable and kind. But how well is that intention fulfilled? This is where the exploration proceeds next:

TEACHER: Let's take a look at how things actually turn out. What are the results of these different strategies?

JAN: If I can, I talk to a close friend of mine. She knows me very well, and she's not fazed by me being in a state.

TEACHER: It sounds like that's really helpful then.

JAN: Yes, it is. I always feel better afterward.

TEACHER: Thank you. (*Draws continuing outward arrow, away from pain.*)

LEYLA: Mine is distraction—I find playing Sudoku on the computer especially good—takes my mind off things.

TEACHER: So, in the short term again, that sounds really helpful.

LEYLA: Yes, that's right.

TEACHER: What about the longer term? When you stop playing, what then?

LEYLA: Well, whatever I was trying not to think about is still there. Sometimes it's worse 'cause I think that I should have been getting on with stuff I have to do, so the game just feels like I am getting behind with my work.

TEACHER: Okay, so helpful in the short term, but maybe not in the long term. (*Draws arrow returning toward pain.*)

WES: Mine is blaming other people.

TEACHER: How does that turn out?

WES: Sometimes I feel a bit better, but sometimes I get into arguments with them. Plus afterward I feel really guilty.

TEACHER: So in the long run, that one doesn't seem to help? In fact, in the long term, it might even make things worse. (*Wes nods.*) Anyone else? (*Collects further examples, then stands back from the board and contemplates it.*) So, what do you make of that?

ROZ: Well, if they worked, we wouldn't be here, would we? (*laughter in the group*)

As these examples show, some reactions are genuinely helpful both in the short term and in the long term. Others, however, even if helpful in the short term, in the long term leave the situation unchanged, and may even make it worse. The essence of the difficulty with automatic, habitual reactions driven by the urgent need to reduce or escape the pain is that they prevent people from seeing clearly what is present and, from a decentered mindful perspective, choosing wisely about how best to respond (see the sidebar on p. 178).

It is important for teachers to approach this exercise with curiosity and an open mind, since what reactions will prove helpful, and how, can be surprising. "Fishing" for unhelpful reactions so as to identify vicious circles can sound like "You're getting it wrong," prompting self-criticism. And even something that on the face of it appears self-evidently unhelpful may turn out to be a lifesaver.

One participant, Al, had a long history of suicidal depression. He was divorced, with a much loved adolescent son. Especially when the boy was staying with his mother, he would try to numb his distress with alcohol. As he put it:

"Before I know where I am, I get stuck in this quagmire in my head. All sorts of thoughts and feelings, whirring round and round. Something goes wrong, and I'm off again. You're such a failure, why can't you get anything right? I get so frustrated and tense, I don't know what to do with myself. Life doesn't seem worth living and maybe, with my son out of the house, would be a good time to get out of it. I think he'd be better off with his mother anyway. That's when I turn to alcohol—a bottle or two and it's all blotted out. When I wake up, I've got a dreadful hangover, but at least I'm alive, I've made it through the night."

He responded to the vicious flower from the perspective of "getting it right":

AL: So what you're saying is that we're doing the wrong thing, we shouldn't be doing these things.

TEACHER: Oh, I'm sorry, no, that's not at all what I wanted to say. Thanks for raising this. At some time, any one of these could have saved your life. So it really isn't a question of throwing them out. It's more a question of adding another string to your bow—a mindful response that allows you to see clearly what's going on, and choose how best to care for yourself.

Here teachers are dealing with the heart of the storm, those crisis moments when pain is extreme. The task is not to take anything away, but rather to offer and embody an alternative: mindful awareness and compassion toward painful experiences, a sense that, in these moments above all, what is most needed is care and kindness, tenderness and gentleness toward the hurt.

STAGE 4: MINDFULNESS AS AN ALTERNATIVE RESPONSE

It often happens that many of the answers to the question about old ways of coping with mental pain fall into two broad categories:

avoidance (e.g., distraction, suppression, intentional numbing) and elaboration (e.g., rumination, worry, arguing with oneself, analyzing). The teacher can summarize and close the "vicious flower" discussion by highlighting these (see Figure 11.3):

> "It's possible to see these reactions as falling into two groups: 'avoidance' and 'entanglement.' [Writes 'avoidance' at one side of the board and 'entanglement' at the other. Draws a horizontal line between them.] What would be examples of avoidance, from our flower? And entanglement? [Gets one or two examples of each.] Unfortunately, neither of these works too well, as we have seen. Quite a few do a good job in the short term, but in the longer term not much changes. Now, the mindfulness you've been practicing for the last 4 weeks is important because it offers an alternative to both of these, especially the practice we did today where you intentionally turned toward something difficult. [Draws an arrow vertically downward from the center of the horizontal line, and writes 'MBCT' at the bottom end.] When you are mindfully aware, you're staying in contact with whatever it is rather than trying to get away from it or control it. [Points to 'avoidance.'] So you have a chance to see clearly what's really going on. And that means you're in a better position to consider how best to care for yourself at that moment. At the same time [pointing to 'elaboration'], you're not getting all tangled up in ruminating about it, or arguing with yourself, or whatever, which adds extra distress to what is already more than distressing enough. What are your reactions to that idea?"

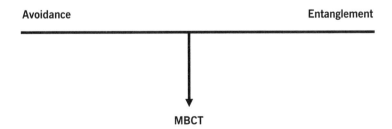

FIGURE 11.3. Avoidance and entanglement: A continuum.

THE TRAFFIC JAM

Many of us have been held up in traffic jams, perhaps on holiday weekends when not only we but the whole population seem to have decided to go out for a drive. In one town in the United Kingdom that is notorious for its traffic jams, a large poster by the side of the road read: *You are not caught in traffic, you are the traffic.*

Trying to *think* your way out of a difficulty is like adding another vehicle to a road already jammed with cars. Consciously choosing not to add more of the same in these moments, perhaps by turning our focus of attention to body or breath or by simply allowing things to be as they are, can allow thoughts to be held (as it were) in a larger space of awareness.

Making Space for the Difficult

Through the "sitting with the difficult" practice and these exercises, we invite participants to disengage from adrenalin-based reactivity and automatic problem-solving processes, even—indeed especially—with unwanted experiences. We invite them simply to pause, to notice this experience just as it is right now, because it is already here. There is nowhere to get to with this process, nothing to change, all that is needed is actively to open to information about how things actually are in this moment. "Turning toward" is thus not a static process but one that, through our attitude and the stance we adopt, acknowledges and allows a direct experiencing of whatever is here, in its entirety.

This mode of approach cannot exist alongside avoidant/fear-based processes in the neural pathways in the brain. As we approach we are fostering attitudes of wonder, curiosity, and friendliness to experiences, whatever they may be, whether externally or internally generated. There is a process of *letting go* of the automatic tendency to strive to be rid of it or to find a speedy resolution, to release old, habitual behaviors and instead invite a willingness to experiment with a different way of being. Through direct personal experience, trust is developed in the safety and value of turning toward the difficult and painful, so that a library of experiential knowledge is created that, however counterintuitive it may seem, offers a new and supportive way to relate to experiences that lead to despair.

How do our participants respond to these invitations?

One participant, Chris, sat forward in her chair as she spoke. She looked surprised and was smiling as she described her experience of being with her pain during the practice during Session 5:

> "I started to feel a pain in my back and straight away noticed that I was cross about it and having angry thoughts about it being there like 'Go away!' and 'Why now, why me?' Then I saw this and imagined making a big container to hold it all—my painful back, my thoughts, and my irritation."

As she said this her arms reached outward to create the shape of a big wide bowl, reaching outward and downward. Her shoulders were low and at ease.

A second participant, John, sat still and steady with a firm, connected base after the practice. He described how his thoughts had rushed along with familiar and emotive content that generally pulled him into their narrative.

> "This time I saw it really clearly and realized that I had a choice. I decided to drop right down into my body [making a sound like a heavy sandbag landing; silence for a few moments]. The thoughts didn't go away but it was like they were a radio playing a long way away. The thoughts could be there without me needing to be involved with what they were telling me."

He gestured the radio he pictured to the right behind him with a large circular movement of his hand. He was showing in this gesture that he wasn't pushing it away but instead allowing it to be just a part of his experience, peripheral to this steady, rooted presence, held in a bigger space.

A third participant, Bethan, said the experience of making space for difficulty felt like a lake she knew in the mountains near her home. She felt the strength of the rock beneath the lake but the vastness of the space that had room for all experiences.

It is not always like this, but simply to hear that it is possible for people—who have had such difficult experiences in the past—to relate to these patterns coming up right now is encouraging. For these participants, making space for experience was adding an additional dimension to that of turning toward. It seems as if a container or space is being created within ourselves that is physically and emotionally large enough and substantial enough to tenderly hold all the elements of this experience, even those that are not welcome and even feel actively threatening.

The nonverbal communications, when these experiences are described, show a steadiness and grounding in the body, especially the lower part of the body, the chest and chin lifting and often the arms opening to show space and a sense of a steady container. No longer is the experience all that is felt, overwhelming attention, but instead there is a process of decentering in order to see the broader view.

Options for the Order of Events in Session 5

When we first were adapting MBCT for people at risk of suicide, we followed the session structure outlined in Table 11.1. However, a helpful alternative arose serendipitously in one 8-week course. Several participants had been unable to attend Session 4 where the long sitting (breath, body, sounds, thoughts, open awareness) was introduced. They had practiced this at home during the week, but had had no opportunity to experience it in the group, together with the reflective space offered by the inquiry. The teacher decided to open the class with the long sitting from Session 4, followed by the practice inquiry and the home practice review, and discovered that experiences of difficulty and a range of reactions to it naturally emerged in the course of this. It then felt completely natural and logical to introduce the new practice, albeit in a somewhat shorter form (20 minutes), focusing on breath, body, and the difficult as we have described earlier. This format then became an alternative option for teachers. Both options are outlined in Table 11.2; what is different in Option 2 is in *italics*.

TABLE 11.2. MBCT for People at Risk of Suicide: Options for the Structure of Session 5

Option 1	Option 2
30- to 40-minute sitting practice (breath; body; exploring difficulty and reactions to difficulty in the body)	*30- to 40-minute sitting practice (breath; body; sounds; thoughts; choiceless awareness)*
Inquiry	Inquiry
Home practice review	Home practice review
	20-minute sitting (breath; body; exploring difficulty and reactions to difficulty in the body)
	Inquiry
Mental pain: The territory of despair • What makes it difficult to bear? • Reactions to pain • Mindful awareness as an alternative to avoidance and entanglement	Mental pain: The territory of despair • What makes it difficult to bear? • Reactions to pain • Mindful awareness as an alternative to avoidance and entanglement
3-minute breathing space (additional instructions) and inquiry	3-minute breathing space (additional instructions) and inquiry
Rumi: "The Guest House"	Rumi: "The Guest House"
Home practice assignment: • Sitting with breath, body, sounds, thoughts, choiceless awareness • 3-minute breathing space three times daily • 3-minute breathing space + additional instructions when notice difficulty	Home practice assignment: • Sitting with breath, body, sounds, thought, choiceless awareness • 3-minute breathing space three times daily • 3-minute breathing space + additional instructions when notice difficulty

Concluding Remarks

So Session 5 was the hardest of all for many highly vulnerable participants, and can create an understandable fear in teachers too. People who are depressed, or fearful of depression and the intensely painful thoughts and emotions that accompany it, will want to create distance from these experiences in whatever ways are possible. As teachers, we are also aiming to teach a sense of creating distance, but in a subtly different way—one that is imbued with a sense of curiosity rather than aversion or pushing away. This approach is about "making space for" rather than "creating distance from"; learning to move close without getting stuck. The experience of "turning toward" encourages this shift in attitude to occur because it allows people to sense how they are relating to the difficult—using the body as a barometer to sense how much they are, in this very moment, "opening to," "softening around," and "dropping in to" what threatens their well-being.

Little by little, people realize that a momentary "slice" of experience never occurs without at least the beginning of an *attitude toward* that experience—in every moment—and that they have a choice: to become aware of such attitudes, to see their consequences, and to *change orientation* to the experience. This change involves beginning to face toward difficult experiences and to become still (rather than moving away), perhaps even to move gently toward them with an attitude of friendly wondering and curiosity, rather than with any intent to change or resolve them.

CHAPTER 12

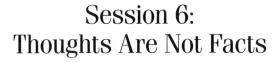

Session 6:
Thoughts Are Not Facts

Session 6

Following Session 5, where difficult situations are turned toward and explored, Session 6 looks more closely at how thoughts contribute to the picture. The syllabus, the intentions of each element, and associated home practices are summarized in Table 12.1.

Working with thoughts is generally acknowledged to be one of the most challenging meditation practices. This difficulty is magnified for vulnerable people when thoughts can feel so toxic and dangerous. Of course, thoughts have been noticed again and again during the program: mind wandering in the raisin and body scan in Session 1; automatic interpretations in the *walking down the street* exercise in Session 2; a component of pleasant and unpleasant experiences in Sessions 3 and 4; the ATQ (negative thinking and the territory of depression) in Session 4; relating to thoughts as we relate to sounds in the guided meditation, also in Session 4; the toxic thoughts and images that are turned toward in Session 5. What is there left to focus on in Session 6?

Whereas the earlier sessions (especially Session 2) focus on thoughts as a major contributor to emotional feelings, Session 6 explores the other side of the vicious circle: how feelings give birth to thoughts. The teacher explores how difficult it can be to see thoughts at all—never mind seeing them as passing mental events; how easily

TABLE 12.1. Week 6: Summary of Practices

Session theme	Practices and exercises	Skills learned	Insights supported by practices	Home practice
Thoughts are not facts Aim: to encourage participants to reduce their identification with thoughts and to begin to relate to thoughts, including difficult thoughts, as mental events.	*Sitting meditation* A meditation in which thoughts form the object of awareness (Audio Track 11[a]). Thoughts are observed arising and passing away, rather than being sought out. This process is supported through the use of metaphors—imagining thoughts as images on a cinema screen, or as clouds passing in the sky, or leaves on a river. Participants are then invited to deliberately bring to mind a difficult thought and to adopt the same attitude of openness and nonjudgmental awareness. If this proves too difficult, because the thoughts that arise are extremely distressing, participants are encouraged to bring awareness to the impact of the thoughts on the body, and to stay with and observe these sensations, before returning to the experience of passing thoughts.	To further develop the ability to stay with difficult thoughts that arise during meditation practice. To practice becoming aware of the bodily responses to difficult thoughts and to attend to these as a form of grounding, rather than resorting to attempting to suppress or challenge the content of difficult thoughts.	It is possible to stay with difficult thoughts rather than engaging in habitual, but unhelpful, reactions. Remaining with difficult thoughts and observing them from a decentered perspective, can, over time, lead to a reduction in their capacity to evoke emotions.	*Shorter guided meditations* Participants are given a series of shorter guided meditations (Audio Tracks 4, 7, 10, and 13) and are encouraged to mix and match these to build up a flexible practice that they can maintain in daily life. Yoga practice and walking meditation can also be incorporated into these routines if participants find them to be helpful. *Breathing spaces* Participants are encouraged to continue using breathing spaces (Audio Tracks 8 and 9) at regular intervals and at times of stress. The breathing space is emphasized as a response that introduces greater choice and flexibility in responding to difficulty.

184

Ambiguous scenarios

Participants are introduced to a further ambiguous scenario—someone being too busy to talk to them—and are asked to explore the different reactions they would have if they had just had a quarrel with someone at work as compared to if they had just had a positive appraisal from their boss.

To take a metacognitive perspective, reflecting on the impact that internal and external contexts have on reactions to events and experiences.

Interpretations of events can be heavily influenced by context and the mental state we bring to the event. Mindful awareness can allow us to see events and their contexts more clearly and as a result increase flexibility of responding.

Relapse signatures

Participants work alone and in groups or pairs to identify their own warning signs for depressive relapse.

To become familiar with one's own warning signs of depressive relapse

---

ᵃAudio recordings of the guided mindfulness meditation practices used in the MBCT program are available to readers for streaming or downloading at www.guilford. com/williams6-materials.

disguised they are: how easy it is to take them personally without realizing what is happening; and how they provide the context for interpretations of other unrelated situations.

> Fiona arrived at the start of Session 6 looking tired and sad. During the class she described having had a challenging week with the family arguments that were a regular feature of her wider family. Comments from members of her family, made in moments of anger, had triggered familiar and painful thoughts for Fiona. The comments they made had been hurtful and she found herself believing what they had said. Their accusations matched her own doubts about herself and mirrored her own self-critical tendency. Fiona recognized that she believed both her family's comments and her own thoughts arising from the arguments: "When it's bad, I feel like a get sucked into a huge whirlpool, lost inside it, spun around by the thoughts and emotions, so disoriented that I can't see my way out."

Here, Fiona feels the strength of the pull of these thoughts and even recognizes the felt sense of being "lost" in them. Talking about this in the class reflected a willingness to consider if these thoughts were indeed facts, even if the emotion felt with them was powerful and the content familiar. However, it was clear that she was easily drawn back into the whirlpool where the experience was very strong. By asking for the support of the group, she could begin to explore new possibilities. Speaking about them in the class, she described finding steadier ground from which to see this painful thinking.

This is how Segal et al. (2013, p. 310) describe this process:

> We can imagine we are in a cinema or theater and simply decide to watch the film or theater of the mind as thoughts come and go on the screen or stage. We can also look out for those *thoughts that seem to "come from behind" in the theater*—like a whisper in the ear from the seat behind (e.g., "This is not going so well"; "There's no point in doing this"; "It's not going to work, so why bother?"; "This pain is killing me"; "I wish this practice would end"; "This is so hard, I'm never going to be any good at it. Why does everything always go wrong?"). These are difficult to see as mental events, for they do not appear on the "stage" we are watching.
>
> So the instructor may point out that some thoughts come from other "places" and that these (to change the analogy) can get "under

the radar" of our practice of "observing thoughts." We may invite participants to think of their theater as having "surround sound"— or if they are imagining themselves sitting on the banks of a river, to imagine that part of the river may also be running behind them, easily missed, but also carrying some leaves in its stream. However, we also point out that this is not easy to do, and it should be practiced for only 3 or 4 minutes at a time in the early stages.

What is happening here is that participants are seeing more clearly that sometimes *thoughts are not seen as mental events because they are "camouflaged" by emotion.* Emotions—strong or weak—can give birth to thoughts and images, like bubbles rising in a simmering pan. Sometimes the most skillful way of dealing with persistent or repetitive thoughts is to "go underneath," to get a sense of what emotions might be giving rise to them.

Now we can see why this step is left until Session 6: it is very helpful to have practiced (in Session 5 and the home practice that follows) noticing what body sensations accompany difficulties. It now becomes possible to deal with negative thoughts and images in the same way: turning attention to the body so as to explore what emotions and accompanying physical sensations are to be found here. This may open up the possibility of discovering new things: for instance, that an angry thought is arising, yes, from anger, but also sadness and fear may be here too. Seeing this more clearly creates a sense of new insight, and also a slight "release" of automatic reactions that have dogged similar situations in the past—a freedom to respond in new ways. We build on this by incorporating *approaching thoughts differently* into the breathing space (Audio Track 9) for the next week (see Teasdale et al., 2014, pp. 161–162).

Seeing Thoughts as Mental Events: The Consequences

Jason began to learn from this practice to recognize that he could now relate to frightening thoughts differently:

> "My boss was giving me feedback this week about a piece of work that I'd done. Some good, some bad . . . but I began to notice the

bad—and then began to have very familiar thoughts about how hopeless I am and how people don't think I'm good at anything. I noticed them quite quickly this time and said to myself that they were just territory of depression thoughts, like we talked about a couple of weeks ago. Then I remembered something you'd said in a previous class about letting the 'thought buses' go past. You don't have to get on a bus just because it stops at the bus stop. I knew that if I got on one of these thought buses they would take me to a very dark place. If I did that it would be just like choosing to get on a bus that I knew was going a very different direction to where I wanted to go."

Jason is describing ways he had discovered of being with these painful and potentially dangerous thought processes through his growing awareness. From such awareness, choices begin to become available. Others in the class responded to this insight. They began to report other instances of how the habitual patterns, even when their pull was very strong, could be held and responded to once they had the courage to pause and turn toward them kindly so that they could be seen clearly.

Relapse Prevention Work

Given that a prime intention of MBCT is to offer participants a means of staying well, or at the least responding differently when depressed mood recurs, it was important as the end of the program approached to consider how to carry new learning into the future. Each participant identifies a form of mindfulness meditation practice that can realistically be used on a continuing basis in the real world. Since the classes cannot guarantee that depression will never occur again—any more than any other treatment approach, whether medical or psychological—space is also given to looking ahead, considering what signs and signals might indicate that all is not well, and how best to respond to them.

In the original program, this information was introduced in Session 7. We felt that, given our participants' intense and speedy reactions to low mood, it would be wise to start the process in Session 6, then build on it in Sessions 7 and 8 (this change has been incorporated into the second edition of the MBCT manual; Segal et al., 2013, pp. 318–230).

We developed two new worksheets, and in Session 6, focused on the first, which was designed to help participants identify personal relapse signatures. (The second, for beginning to identify how best to *respond* when signs of possible relapse occurred, will be introduced in Session 7). The worksheet was introduced during a short contemplation, following a breathing space. A completed example is shown in Figure 12.1.

RESPONDING WISELY TO UNHAPPINESS AND DEPRESSION (1)

Seeing Clearly *(noticing the first signs of depression)*

This worksheet offers an opportunity to increase your awareness of what happens for you when depression appears. The aim is, carefully and with curiosity, to investigate the thoughts, feelings, body sensations, and patterns of behavior that tell you that your mood is starting to drop.

What triggers depression for you?
- Triggers can be external (things that happen to you), or internal (e.g., thoughts, feelings, memories, concerns).
- Look out for small triggers as well as large ones—sometimes something that appears quite trivial can spark a downward mood spiral.

Arguments with my husband

Too much to do at work

Being tired or unwell

What sort of thoughts run through your mind when you first feel your mood dropping?

Here I go again. Why can't I get a handle on this?

I'm just useless at dealing with any kind of stress.

Every time, I think that's the last time, and then here it is again.

What's the point?

What emotions arise?

Disappointed, frustrated

Guilt for letting it happen

Hopelessness

(continued)

FIGURE 12.1. Participant worksheet, Session 6.

What happens in your body?

Sinking feeling, knot in stomach

Tension, especially in my neck and shoulders

Weighed down

What do you do, or feel like doing?

Cut myself off from everybody

Staying in bed with the duvet over my head

Drink too much, keep going with coffee and sugar

Think about putting an end to it

Are there any old habits of thinking or behavior that might unwittingly keep you stuck in depression (e.g., ruminating, trying to suppress or turn away from painful thoughts and feelings, struggling with them instead of accepting and exploring them)?

Trying to get away from the feelings, however I can, to the point of thinking of offing myself.

Alcohol—feel better in the short term, but doesn't really help. More likely to get into arguments.

Being horrible to myself—constant criticism and put-downs.

FIGURE 12.1. (continued)

Participants began this work in the class, and then after a brief inquiry continued to reflect on and elaborate it during the following week. To facilitate this practice, the teacher might say:

"It's important to keep the worksheet somewhere where you can easily find it. Holding the questions at the back of your mind, notice what else occurs to you as the week goes on, and jot it down. Another thing people often find really useful is to tell someone who knows them well, and who they trust, what they're doing. This is because people who know us well can often tell when all is not well some time before we become aware of it, when the signs and signals are still quite subtle. So if you have someone like that, it could be really useful to ask him or her what he or she notices when your mood begins to dip, and perhaps think together about how he or she might most helpfully respond if the signs appear."

Here we explicitly turn toward the ultimate intention of the program: staying well after depression. Just as previous practices have taught participants that awareness is the first step toward choice, and the importance of turning toward what is most difficult and challenging, so here we encourage participants to turn toward the possibility of future depressions, with the intention of cultivating awareness as a prelude to responding wisely when early signals appear.

Concluding Remarks

Whereas in Session 2 the influence of thinking on feelings is highlighted, here in Session 6 the reciprocal influence of mood on thought is brought into focus, how particular moods "give birth to" particular patterns of thought. Echoing this pattern, we turn explicitly toward the future, inviting participants to cultivate decentered awareness of their personal "relapse signatures"—the thoughts, emotions, body sensations, and behaviors that tell them that all is not well. Gentle, kind—and courageous—awareness offers a new place to stand steadily when the internal dialogue becomes powerful and mood begins to shift.

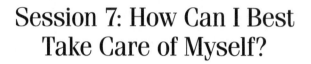

CHAPTER 13

Session 7: How Can I Best Take Care of Myself?

Session 7 follows the format of standard MBCT. The syllabus, the intentions and of each element, associated home practices are summarized in Table 13.1.

Activity and Mood

The sitting practice at the start of the class (Audio Track 11) is based on that used in Session 4, but allows many longer silences for participants to do the practice for themselves. The practice review is followed as usual by a home practice review, and then by an exercise in which participants generate a list of activities they do on a typical working day (exactly how many the teacher invites them to call to mind depends on the time available—it might be 12–15, or perhaps 6–8). This is how Segal et al. (2013, p. 338) introduce the practice:

> Take a moment to bring to mind what you do during a typical working day. If you spend much of your day apparently doing the same thing, try breaking the activities down into smaller parts: talking to colleagues, e-mailing, making coffee, filing, word processing, eating lunch. And what about evenings and weekends? What sort of things

do you find yourself doing then? Make a list in your mind's eye or on paper. Now see if you can see what things on the list lift your mood, give you energy, nourish you. And what things on your list are things that dampen your mood or drain your energy?

The aim is to encourage participants to reflect, first individually, then in pairs, and finally in the class as a whole what activities nourish and what activities deplete them. They may find it helpful to place a letter *N* next to those activities that feel nourishing and a *D* against those that feel depleting. Working with these, the teacher then introduces a discussion of how to work to increase the availability of nourishment and deal skillfully with depleting activities and situations, exploring the differences between different types of nourishment: mastery (M) activities and pleasure (P) activities. These draw on the decades of research that has gone into cognitive and behavioral theory and therapy for depression and are critical aspects of the teaching in Session 7. Many subtle teaching issues need to be explored and communicated interactively, rather than didactically, and we find that many mindfulness teachers who are not familiar with or at ease with cognitive or behavioral traditions find it difficult to understand their significance fully. The issues are carefully laid out in Teasdale et al. (2014; pp. 171–179) so we will not explore them further here (see also Segal et al., 2103, pp. 339–343). The activities exercise may be followed by a breathing space, at the end of which there is an invitation to bring to mind ways, however small, of changing the balance of nourishment and depletion in favor of nourishment.

Preparing for the Future

When this exercise is complete, the teacher returns to the *Responding Wisely (1)* worksheet participants have done at home (Figure 12.1). It is first discussed in pairs, and then in the group as a whole. There is usually a great deal of discussion about the triggers for low mood that are commonly shared between participants, and those that are unique to each individual. Then the second worksheet is introduced (see Figure 13.1):

TABLE 13.1. Week 7: Summary of Practices

Session theme	Practices and exercises	Skills learned	Insights supported by practices	Home practice
How can I best take care of myself? Aim: To explore how awareness can be used to guide skillful action.	*Sitting meditation (Audio Track 11[a])* This follows the format outlined above.	To further develop the ability to attend to, stay with, and be open to experiences as they arise during meditation practice.		*Self-directed practice* Participants choose from all the formal meditation practices they have learned and settle on one or more that will be realistic to use on a daily basis after the course is over.
	Relapse signatures Participants work in groups to discuss what to do when relapse threatens.	To see shared and unique triggers, and how easy it is to become enmeshed in the mood they create; and to see what they might do to take care of themselves in these situations (not forgetting the *crisis card* they completed at the preclass interview).	An awareness of the differences between reacting and responding wisely at times of low mood.	*Breathing spaces* Participants continue to use scheduled and spontaneous breathing spaces (Audio Tracks 8 and 9) to integrate mindfulness into daily life and as a means of *taking action* to respond wisely to challenging experiences.
		To reflect on the consequences of different activities for mood and well-being.		*Relapse prevention planning* Participants elaborate their relapse prevention plan and include information about other people who may be able to provide help or support.
		To use a breathing space at times of low mood to explore whether the wisest response to a difficult situation is to adopt mindful awareness of ongoing experience or to take skillful action.		

194

Reflection on daily activities

Participants list daily activities and divide them into those that lift mood, give energy, and are nourishing and those that dampen mood and drain energy.

Working in small groups participants explore how to increase the occurrence of nourishing activities (including very small events) and reduce the occurrence of depleting activities, while holding difficult aspects of their lives in mind, rather than simply trying to avoid them.

Participants then reflect on nourishing activities identifying those that lift mood by providing a sense of mastery and those that do so by providing a sense of pleasure. They reflect on how best to use what they have discovered—for example, taking a breathing space, reflecting on how things are in the moment, and making a conscious choice about how to respond.

If appropriate to deliberately increase the occurrence of activities that lift mood and provide a sense of mastery or pleasure at times of low mood.

An awareness of the balance of nourishing and depleting activities in our lives and how this can be modified without simply avoiding difficulties.

[a]Audio recordings of guided mindfulness meditation practices used in the MBCT program are available to readers for streaming or downloading at *www.guilford.com/williams6-materials*.

"Let us consider how you might most helpfully respond when you notice these triggers or early warning signs of depression. Let's begin with a breathing space. [Leads breathing space.] And as you sit with breath and body, allowing these questions to resonate in your awareness, and noticing what arises in the mind. [Reads questions from worksheet, with pauses for answers to arise in the mind of participants.] And now opening your eyes, and turning to the sheet. Noting down whatever came to mind as you contemplated the questions."

When the writing dies down, the teacher can invite participants to work further together in pairs, sharing ideas and experiences and helping one another to refine the picture of early warning signals and how best to respond to them. This work can once again become part of home practice, and a final visit to the sheets can be part of Session 8. It is important to make it clear that such summaries and plans are never complete because it is impossible at a particular moment to predict everything that will happen or to identify everything that might help. So it is useful for participants to recognize that discovering how best to stay well is a continuing exercise in treating yourself with wisdom and kindness, and learning to respond to new challenges with openness, curiosity, and compassion.

Concluding Remarks

We have deliberately been economical in describing this session, as the procedures are well described in the second edition of MBCT for depression and in the workbook. For those who are vulnerable to suicide, the preparation to respond wisely to downturns of mood when they inevitably come is extremely important. Each participant will have prepared a crisis card at an earlier stage (see pp. 88–89), and this is an opportunity as the program comes to an end to link back the learning of Session 7 to that card with its list of names of helpful people to contact. Teachers are always aware of thoughts that arise to undermine intentions, and it may be particularly useful to spend time toward the end of Session 7 examining (in pairs and with the class as

RESPONDING WISELY TO UNHAPPINESS AND DEPRESSION (2)

Caring for yourself when you notice the first signs of depression

On the handout in Session 6, you wrote down what triggers downward spirals in mood for you, and what signs you notice that your mood is dropping (e.g., thoughts, feelings, body sensations). On this sheet, we consider how you might skillfully respond when you find yourself in this position. It may be helpful to look back over your course handouts, to remind yourself of what you have done and see if you have discovered anything that might help.

In the past, what have you noticed that helped when you were becoming depressed?

Talking to somebody, especially Mom or a close friend

Going to the GP—I don't necessarily want pills, but it's good to speak to someone professional and uninvolved in my life

Making myself do something I might enjoy, especially getting out into the countryside

Taking it slow

Reminding myself of the good things in my life

What might be a skilful response to the pain of depression? How could you respond to the turmoil of thoughts and feelings without adding to it (including what you have learned in the classes)?

Keep using the breathing space to put on the pause button when things are getting too much.

Do the lying-down stretches every day, even if it feels it won't make a difference.

Be kind to myself—how would I treat another person I cared about who was feeling this way?

Read the course folder, and my own notes—remind myself of everything I've learned and how things changed for me.

How can you best care for yourself at this difficult and painful time (e.g. things that would soothe you, activities that might nourish you, people you might contact, small things you could do to respond wisely to distress)?

Have a warm bath—get something special that smells good so I've got it ready.

Do some gardening—it's good to get my hands dirty and be with growing things.

Cuddle the cat.

(continued)

FIGURE 13.1. Participant worksheet, Session 7.

Ring up Sue—she'll make me laugh and feel good.

Tell Mom how I'm feeling.

If I need to, accept that medication may help take the edge off it.

If I need to back out and have a duvet day, that's okay—just make sure it's a conscious decision, not me on automatic pilot.

Do something physical—go for a swim or a walk.

Go back to doing a long meditation every day—and don't be hard on myself if I don't manage it.

BE KIND TO MYSELF. EVEN IF I DON'T FEEL I DESERVE IT

It may be helpful to remind yourself that what you need at times of difficulty is no different from what you have already practiced many times throughout the course.

FIGURE 13.1. *(continued)*

a whole) what things (thoughts feelings, circumstances) will stop them taking wise action. This might be explicitly linked to what the class did in Session 1, preparing themselves for the difficulty in doing home practice by anticipating what barriers might arise.

The sense of the imminent ending of the 8-week program is palpable, so looking forward can be both important and poignant at this point. The session's focus on what will support and nourish connects directly with life beyond the course. The ordinariness of nourishing activities (savoring a cup of coffee first thing in the morning, making time to walk in nature) makes them accessible to all. There is no need to search for special events; the everyday, chosen with wise and mindful awareness, is enough to nourish body and mind. Sometimes simply *doing* an activity is important, even if—especially if—motivation or mood are low. At other times, what is most important is to stay present to an activity, whatever it is. This is a dynamic and responsive process of noticing and responding, moment by moment, offering care and support as experience unfolds. This is mindful awareness in action.

CHAPTER 14

Session 8: Maintaining and Extending New Learning

Session 8

Session 8 follows closely the pattern of *Mindfulness-Based Cognitive Therapy for Depression* (Segal et al., 2013), so we will not go into further detail here. The syllabus and the intentions of each element are summarized in Table 14.1 (the only home practice is what participants themselves decide to pursue after the end of the course).

Following a return to the body scan (see Segal et al., 2013, pp. 365–378) and a very brief enquiry, the relapse action plans are revisited.

Participants discover from each other what it is they have decided to put on their responding wisely action plan (see Session 7, Chapter 13). During the week, they may have had time to discuss the worksheet with a family member or close friend, and it may be helpful to check in with each other—in pairs or small groups—to see what aspect of their plans have changed in the light of these discussions.

To sum up the relapse prevention work, we asked participants to return to sitting in silence, focusing on the breath and body for a few moments, and to allow answers to this question to arise in the mind:

"From the work that you've done, if there was just one thing to help you stay well which you would want above all to remember, what would that one thing be?"

TABLE 14.1. Week 8: Summary of Practices

Session theme	Practices and exercises	Skills learned	Insights supported by practices	Home practice
Maintaining and extending new learning Maintaining balance in life is helped by regular mindfulness practice.	*Body scan (Audio Track 3ᵃ)* As described earlier.	To focus attention on different body sensations. To remain open to whatever arises in awareness.	Experiences and responses to the practice may have changed over time in the light of new learning.	Whatever participants themselves decide to do following the course.
Good intentions can be strengthened by linking the practice with positive reasons for taking care of yourself.	*Reflection* Participants reflect either alone or in pairs, on their initial intentions in coming to classes, what they have learned, and potential obstacles for continuing practice.	Participants are encouraged to aim for daily practice, even if only for very brief periods of time, and are introduced to the idea of beginner's mind—that it is always possible to restart practice, even after a long break.		
	Feedback Participants give written feedback on their experiences in the class.			
	Closing Final sitting followed by well-wishing for self and each other.			

ᵃAudio recordings of guided mindfulness meditation practices used in the MBCT program are available to readers for streaming or downloading at *www.guilford. com/williams6-materials*.

Answers can be shared in the large group. Here are some examples given by participants in our classes:

"Don't let yourself pretend it's not happening, do something NOW."

"Be kind to yourself."

"Continue to practice."

"There's a big difference between 'I am useless' and 'Here it is, thinking I am useless.'"

"Make nourishing activities part of everyday life—and especially when you don't feel good."

"There are people who care for you. Don't be afraid to ask them for help."

"Use the breathing space."

After this, it was important in the closing session to allow time for feedback on what had been learned and on how to sustain future learning. Reflection was introduced through a short meditation (see the sidebar below), in which questions were allowed to "drop into" the silence. What came out of these reflections was little different from the ending of many other mindfulness classes: that mindfulness was challenging for all involved. It took courage for the participants to take the opportunities to turn toward the sometimes challenging and painful material that could arise in and between classes. There was a sense of a "work in progress"—of more exploration to be done. Despite this, there were many stories indicating to all that this approach had

---

MEDITATION AND REFLECTION
(5 MINUTES ALONE, THEN 10 MINUTES IN PAIRS)

Sitting with breath, then allowing these questions to be here:

"Why did you come?"

"What have you discovered?"

"What obstacles did you encounter?"

"How did you deal with them?"

"What do you most wish to take away with you?"

the potential to be transformational, offering a new, relevant, and radically different way to relate to painful experience. Participants showed by their attitude and their stories that they were starting to build the foundation to hold toxic mind states more tenderly, kindly, and confidently, and to take care of themselves.

Some participants described feeling upset that they hadn't learned about this approach years ago when it made so much sense to them now. To discover that difficult experience itself cannot destroy you was often named as a powerful learning through the MBCT course; a new discovery of resilience and strength. Once experienced, it made sense (in a way that it had not before) to turn toward and make space for even the darkest experiences.

Concluding Remarks

In these chapters we have explored specific issues that came up when offering mindfulness to highly vulnerable people, and the changes we made to the 8-week MBCT program in the interests of helping them to benefit fully from what it might offer. As we said, plans to deal skillfully with overwhelming difficulties and the tendency to relapse back into are always in the background. It is simply not possible to predict everything that may happen in the future. Mindfulness teaching is about staying open, as much as it is about implementing a curriculum—and this is true for participants as well as for teachers. Encountering future challenges is part of an ongoing learning process, a continuing independent exploration of the habits of the mind, the changing flow of emotion and sensation, and the developing capacity to respond even to future depression and despair with warmth, curiosity, and (above all) compassion.

The theme at the heart of this work is how to respond wisely to pain and distress that seem intolerable. The teachers' own practice and clear understanding of suicidal depression and the processes that create and maintain it were crucial to trust in the process for this vulnerable group—and the weekly cosupervision group was a hugely important factor in allowing us to see new perspectives and not to lose heart when dealing with the most difficult situations. We were taken back again and again to the foundations that had been laid by our own teachers and our own training. We realized that thorough basic training in how to teach MBCT is essential, but not, on its own, enough. The need for ongoing continuing development and support in responding to the specific issues that arose for people at such high risk was also paramount. We will return to these issues in Chapter 16. First, in Chapter 15, we give a sense of how the whole program unfolded, by focusing on the experience of one participant.

CHAPTER 15

How Does MBCT
Enable Transformation?

Jane's Story

For people who have suffered substantial adversity and are as a result vulnerable to depression and suicidality, the pain of being mindful of present moment experience can be extreme. The program itself brings participants closely in touch with the very patterns that they spend the rest of their lives working to avoid. How does the teaching process support this delicate and difficult work?

In previous chapters in Part II, we have outlined the assessment procedures we used to sharpen our awareness of the risks facing our participants and described the changes we made to the preclass interview to deal with the real issue of helping them to engage with the program. We have described the changes we made to the program itself, with a view to meeting the needs of our vulnerable participants more effectively, and discussed the themes and issues that commonly emerge during the process of following the 8-week MBCT course with people at high risk. In this chapter, we show how these changes and themes unfolded in the experience of a particular participant and the group she was a part of, with a particular focus on how the teacher guides the interactive and inquiry aspects of the teaching.

Inquiry in MBCT

There is a well-developed practitioner literature that describes the process and principles underpinning inquiry in MBCT and MBSR (R.

Crane, 2009; Felder, Dimidjian, & Segal, 2012; McCown et al., 2010; Santorelli, 1999; Segal et al., 2013). An inquiry sequence is described in this literature as occurring in the following generic way.

Following the meditation practice, the teacher begins a conversation by asking participants what they noticed during the practice. They do this to encourage reflection and exploration on their experience; work together through *dialogue about* these observations to find out what is being discovered; and *link* these observations and discoveries to the learning themes of the program. Inquiry aims to reveal and bring into conscious awareness automated and unrecognized habits and patterns of thinking and feeling and to make known some of the properties of thoughts and feelings.

The manner of attending to experience, the teacher, *and* the relational process are all thus aiming to offer an embodiment of the attitudinal qualities of mindfulness. It is suggested that this supports participants to internalize a mindful way of relating to experience that includes increased levels of self-compassion, reduced levels of cognitive reactivity, and the development of a capacity to "allow," rather than problem-solve, whatever experience is present in the moment.

That is how it works in theory, but how does it feel in practice? Let's turn to the 8-week MBCT course we taught, and travel alongside one participant, Jane, as she journeys through the program, occasionally drawing on other participants's experiences as well. We shall especially focus on how inquiry helped Jane to explore, discover, and make changes in the ways she approached her experience and her life.

Jane's Journey through the MBCT Course*

Jane is 48 and works in a travel agency. She lives alone, but her grown-up daughter, her partner, and 3-year-old granddaughter live nearby. She was brought up by her grandmother following the sudden, unexpected death of her mother when she was 4. Her father had severe mental health problems, was in touch with her only erratically during her childhood, and now remains a distant figure in her life. Her grandmother

---

*All of the patient examples in the extended dialogues in this chapter are fictions or composites or are sufficiently disguised that identification would not be possible.

looked after her well physically but was emotionally distant, and Jane was a shy, anxious, and hypervigilant child. She experienced her first episode of depression after the birth of her daughter when she was 20. Now she repeatedly ruminates on the loss of this time with her baby. She feels she has let her daughter down and experiences waves of associated guilt, sadness, and regret. This is further compounded by the strong waves of suicidal ideas and impulses that accompanied the recurring depressions that followed this first episode. Jane knows how much pain she would cause her daughter if she ever acted on these ideas and strongly condemns herself for "even thinking about being so selfish." She is well respected at work because she sets high standards for herself and is immensely productive. She works hard to keep her life in order by being highly organized, taking pride in her appearance, and keeping her house and garden meticulously tidy. We will now follow Jane's journey through the classes one by one, starting with the preclass interview.

Preclass Interview

During the preclass interview the teacher supported Jane to "unpack" the patterns that led into and maintained her depression, by investigating the specific sequence of processes that had led to her last episode 18 months earlier. Jane described how she always worked to keep herself busy because she was better when she "didn't have time to think." Over a period of several months she had pushed herself particularly hard because she had (for "no particular reason") been plagued by particularly strong waves of self-condemning and critical thoughts. When she ran out of things "to do" she had exercised long and hard. These strategies had kept her mood from slipping down for some time, but at a certain point she was overcome with physical exhaustion and illness and was forced to stop. She took sick time at work and isolated herself at home. At this point she became overwhelmed by the force and toxicity of her thoughts. Her mood rapidly cascaded down and she was swept into an episode of depression.

The teacher enabled Jane to look at her experience alongside a wider formulation of how depression is understood to be triggered and perpetuated. This helped her to understand how rumination and avoidance (both behavioral and experiential avoidance) were implicated in triggering and maintaining her depression. The teacher shared the diagram in Figure 15.1 as they explored this issue together.

Enabling participants to connect to this wider understanding is an important aspect of the preclass interview. Through this, they begin to see the intention behind the seemingly risky and outrageous idea of turning toward the very aspects of experience that have caused such immense pain in the past. Jane could see the logic behind the process because she knew that the strategies she was using to cope with her mental pain worked for a while but were unsustainable, and that these strategies stood between her and the possibility of taking pleasure in her life. She was also, however, very wary, because she knew from experience that this was deeply dangerous territory and the consequences of it going wrong were drastic. She was highly motivated to find a way that might offer her longer-term relief. The rationale for the program made enough sense to her to convince her that this was an investment worth making.

The teacher and Jane explored these themes together, and worked out strategies that would enable Jane to feel supported and held while she undertook this tender and difficult work. This included filling out the crisis card so that Jane had specific sources of support identified (see Chapter 5); agreeing together that Jane would initiate contact with the teacher outside the sessions if she needed to talk or was feeling vulnerable, and that similarly the teacher would contact Jane if she was concerned. Jane also agreed to talk with her daughter to let her know that she was undertaking the course and that this might be a difficult time. This in itself was a significant step in a new direction: her tendency was to present an "I can cope" message to the world even when she felt despairing inside.

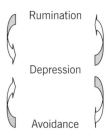

FIGURE 15.1. Vicious circles of rumination and avoidance: both maintain depressed mood.

Session 1: Awareness and Automatic Pilot

Ten days later, along with seven other participants, Jane arrived for Session 1 of the MBCT course. She felt on edge and anxious and sat near the door. The teacher had told her in the preclass interview that the program would offer repeated invitations to investigate aspects of experience that she usually turned away from. Logically, this made sense to Jane—but in practice as she sat there in the class it felt like she was taking a big risk. She had been depression-free for the last 12 months and was fearful that bringing her experience of depression to mind would trigger "dangerous" thoughts.

Jane was a confident speaker in her working context but tried as far as possible in her life to keep her experiences with depression hidden from others. She felt anxious about sharing what brought her to the class and what she was hoping for, first with one other participant and then with the group. However, there was also some relief inherent in hearing others describing experiences she could recognize in herself. Her sense of safety and belonging began to develop as she connected with the group.

During the inquiry after the raisin practice, Jane strongly connected with the theme of automatic pilot—how she rushed around, distracted herself, and so disconnected from immediate experience, with her mind traveling off on trains of association. She could see how she conducted much of the practical activity of her days on autopilot, so it made sense that the activity of her mind might also be driven by habitual automatic patterns. Jane knew that she had an active mind but had not previously seen this as a process over which she had any influence. It was the first time in her life that she had deliberately chosen to notice the detail of this activity. She felt too vulnerable to lie down for the body scan, so chose to sit in a chair. In the inquiry following the practice Jane and the teacher had this exchange:

JANE: I found it really frustrating.

TEACHER: Frustrating.

JANE: My stomach was churning and my heart was pounding a lot of the time. I was thinking of all the things I could be doing, what I'm going to get when I go shopping later. I was dying for you to end; I kept thinking "When is this going to finish?"

TEACHER: Yes . . . so your attention was taken up a lot of the time with thoughts about how long this is, how I don't want to be doing this, how I've got so many other things I could be doing.

The teacher is acknowledging Jane's experience and then highlighting the "phenomenon" of the thinking mind. This invites a shift from aversion to approach-orientated curiosity.

JANE: Absolutely—you got to the lower back and I was thinking oh my god we are only half way there! (*Shared group laughter; teacher looks around, nonverbally acknowledging the recognition of a shared experience.*)

TEACHER: And does any of this feel familiar to you—these sorts of ways of thinking?

JANE: Yes. (*Shared group laughter again.*)

The lightness of shared affiliative laughter in these moments is important. It is a way of coming together to see "our" patterns of mind; it supports a decentered perspective and recognition of the shared (rather than personal) nature of the phenomena that are being observed. Seeing this is an important factor in developing greater compassion for yourself and others—it becomes clear that these patterns are part of the common vulnerability of being human. There is tremendous power in hearing each other's experiences spoken out loud. People see how natural it is not to judge others for having these experiences, so there is a loosening of the tendency to judge themselves.

The teacher then offered to the whole group some teaching themes that emerged out of this exchange with Jane. To support this shift from personal exploration into highlighting general themes, the teacher shifted into the use of "we" and "us" and turned to make eye contact with the whole group. She highlighted how what shows up in the meditation practice is no different from what shows up in our everyday life. The difference is that we have the opportunity in the practice to begin first to see clearly and later to experiment with new ways of working with these familiar thoughts. When they show up in everyday life, we are too busy to begin to see these patterns for what they are. It is a challenging process, but also rich with potential because we can begin to recognize them and explore new ways to work with them.

The themes that come up in practice have a historical dimension—for Jane, the particular patterns of thinking were created through the circumstances of her childhood and had over time become established as habit patterns. In classes, there is kindly acknowledgment of the force of these thoughts, but attention is predominantly placed on how to discover new ways to work with them in the present moment.

Later, the teacher widened the relevance of the theme of challenge to the whole group, and invited them to move into pairs for a few minutes to share together any challenges that they anticipated might crop up in relation to the home practice over this next week. Priming participants to see difficulty as part of the process, rather than an unwanted barrier, is particularly important for this group who, because of their history, are particularly sensitized to withdraw from painful thoughts and emotions (see C. Crane & Williams, 2010). The message that challenge and pain are workable is being conveyed simultaneously on a number of levels. One is the explicit content of the conversation. Another is the teacher's capacity to be at ease and to evenly, warmly, and nonjudgmentally receive all reactions to the practice.

> A mindfulness approach acknowledges that many patterns of mind may come from adversity experiences at an early age; but it does not investigate the origins of these patterns themselves. Rather it focuses on how they are affecting reactions to events in the present.

The teacher invited the group to share some of the themes that had been discussed in the pairs about expected challenges. These included finding the time, finding a space in the house, and working with difficult thoughts and emotions that might come up in the practice. The key message was that the practice is not about trying to create any particular feeling, so there cannot be a "wrong" practice experience. The intention was to support seeing more clearly and getting interested in what was already here. To support motivation and encourage engagement with the practice, the teacher went further by making the connection between depression prevention and the work of noticing thoughts in the practice more explicit. She used Jane's experience as a springboard for this by pointing out that all of the thoughts that she described having during the body scan were "wanting things to be different" sort of thoughts and these tend to elicit painful emotions. The intention of this exploration is to see if it is possible to be more at ease with how things are, however they are.

Session 2: Living in Our Heads

The group met a week later for Session 2. Following the body scan at the start of the session and the inquiry on this, the teacher made space for an exploration of how participants had experienced doing the body scan at home during the week. Jane and the teacher had this interaction:

> JANE: I struggled with it.
> TEACHER: Ah—so would you mind if we explore this a little?

Depending on the "reading" of the participant's nonverbal cues, it can be important to explicitly ask permission before moving into an investigation together.

> JANE: That's fine—when I did the body scan the first time, by the end of it I couldn't move out of my bed and then when I stood up I was just like jelly. I didn't like it. So a lot of days I didn't do it. But I did spend more time lying in bed, leaving the window open and listening to the birds, the cars, and the hustle and bustle of every day.
> TEACHER: And how does it feel to do that?

Jane has shared both her avoidance of the practice following a difficult experience, and some experiences of intentionally pausing to notice more. The teacher chooses to initially direct the inquiry to these.

> JANE: Nice.
> TEACHER: Is that something new?

In each teaching moment there are choices. The teacher could have chosen here to unpack "nice" in terms of its phenomenology of sensations, thoughts, and emotions. However, guided by the way the participant is already communicating her sense of newness to this experience by her emphasis on the word "nice," the teacher follows the participant and makes the choice to explore how experience feels different when we pay attention to it.

> JANE: Oh yes, I don't do that usually! And then I went for a shower afterward and really felt the water [nonverbal communication of the pleasure of the experience].
>
> TEACHER: Ahh—so really making choices to do pleasurable things and noticing your experience.
>
> JANE: I've been trying to notice different things, new things this week.
>
> TEACHER: So you've had a very conscious intention to notice more. How has it felt to do that?
>
> JANE: I realize how much I usually don't see. I miss out.
>
> TEACHER: Ah, yes.

There was a quiet pause in the room at that point. Sometimes it feels intuitively appropriate to simply acknowledge and affirm participants' experience by giving it space, rather than moving into inquiry. Here there was a sense of poignancy related to the loss of connection with experience. The teacher subsequently moved back to the theme that Jane had introduced about not liking the feeling of being so relaxed after the body scan.

> TEACHER: So when you did do the body scan I am curious about the feeling you described that you couldn't move afterward. What did that feel like?
>
> JANE: Like a stone.
>
> TEACHER: Heavy.
>
> JANE: Yes and it was warm and tingly—it was just so funny. I couldn't get up. It's not me to just chill out in bed. I'm awake at six in the morning—on the go.
>
> TEACHER: So you felt heavy, warm, tingly—was this right through the whole of your body or in particular places?
>
> JANE: The whole of me.
>
> TEACHER: And were there any emotions or thoughts that came along with these sensations?

JANE: I got really panicky.

TEACHER: Was that at a particular point or all the way through?

JANE: It was at the end—I felt okay while I was doing it—I was just doing it. Then at the end your voice stopped and I suddenly felt how heavy I was and I thought "I can't move."

TEACHER: It is really great how you are noticing your experience here. So you were just rolling with it, feeling okay and then at the end you had this feeling of being a bit stuck there lying down

The teacher affirmed the participant's skills in noticing the different aspects of her experience. Notice how the inquiry is supporting Jane to take her mind back to this *specific* moment—a moment of acute entrapment—to describe her actual experience, and to "unpack" it in terms of physical sensations (starting here because this is where Jane started), and how these influenced thoughts and emotions.

JANE: Yes—sort of trapped.

TEACHER: Trapped?

JANE: Yes—really weird. I didn't like getting so relaxed—I felt out of control. I felt as though I couldn't move.

TEACHER: And your thinking mind started up saying "I don't like this, I can't move"?

JANE: Yes.

TEACHER: And could you move?

JANE: Well yes—but I felt weird—jelly-like.

TEACHER: Ah, so your thoughts were saying you couldn't move but when you tried to move you discovered that you could?

JANE: I guess—yes.

TEACHER: But this feeling of being relaxed was a bit unusual, a bit odd and your thinking mind started to judge it . . . so it is interesting for us all to notice (*turning to the whole group*) how our ideas about our experience can be quite different from the actuality of our experience.

Notice here how the teacher pauses in the midst of an inquiry with one participant to highlight to the wider group themes that are universally relevant learning points.

> TEACHER: (*turning back to Jane*) And how did you feel emotionally when your thoughts were saying "I can't move"?
>
> JANE: Panicky, sort of scared.
>
> TEACHER: And do you have a sense of what that felt like in your body?
>
> JANE: A sort of rush of hot up through me. (*gesturing with hand around trunk of body*)
>
> TEACHER: And anything else?
>
> JANE: My heart going bang bang here. (*gesturing by patting her hand on her chest*)
>
> TEACHER: So this is really good noticing . . . you have been noticing a lot this week how our experience changes when we pay attention. You have had some really pleasant experiences of noticing things that you usually miss. Here though the "newness" of feeling so relaxed triggered thoughts about being out of control, and strong sensations and emotions in your body.

The experience had been so aversive to Jane that she had not done the body scan during the week at home since. Like others in the group, she has a heightened vigilance to internal experience that is perceived as threatening. Although for many the feeling of being relaxed is pleasurable, for Jane it is associated with a sense of loss of control. With her childhood history of loss and lack of emotional acknowledgment, she learned from an early age that she could get some distance from the intensity of her emotions and thoughts by keeping a tight rein on their expression. When her "guard" is down through becoming relaxed, the fear of being overwhelmed is intense. Her main strategy to stay in control was to keep physically tight and to keep her mind distracted by engaging in activity. When these strategies were interrupted, a sense of entrapment emerged with associated feelings of fear.

Ultimately, mindfulness practice teaches us that we are not in control of our thoughts, sensations, and emotions, but that we can learn to influence what happens next by how we relate to them. The teacher explored with Jane how she could modulate her engagement with the practice so that she could choose when to step forward and experiment with new but challenging possibilities, and when to step back into familiar territory. It is important to acknowledge that distraction is a valid strategy and that this work is about expanding the repertoire of strategies, not about taking away options, as we discussed in Chapter 11.

> The work of mindfulness is about expanding the repertoire of strategies, not about taking away options.

Following this conversation Jane, the teacher, and the rest of the group (who were also working with similar experiences) explored how in practical ways they might find a helpful balance between moving into the challenge of the practice, and at the same time keeping open the valid option of moving back into familiar strategies. The analogy of learning to swim is sometimes used. If you had never been in the water before you would initially sit on the side and kick your legs with the water. After a while you might get in and feel the water over your whole body. You would then gradually build up the skills to swim—but always knowing that you could return to the edge and climb out. Here the theme was anchored to the specific example of what to do when the thought "I can't do this" came up before or during the practice (Jane identified this as her predominant thought since she had experienced her disquieting relaxation). This was connected to the theme of the session—how the chatter of our mind controls our reactions to everyday life and how, without us realizing it, our thoughts propel us into action or prevent action we might otherwise take. Participants are invited as a first step to notice the thought as a thought, and then to tune into sensations in the body. There is an invitation to move away from judgment and into being attentive and curious about experience. So the invitation is to experiment with "pressing the pause button" rather than immediately acting on the thought, redirecting attention to sensations in the body, and then making a more conscious and informed decision about whether to stay with the practice or to step back—and, whichever choice is made, to stay in touch with experience with a particular focus on sensations in the body.

During this inquiry a number of learning processes were in action. Jane and the group were:

- Being trained in a process of tracking and inquiring into the specifics of experience.
- Seeing that learning comes straight out of the immediacy of this experience.
- Acknowledging experience as it is and by so doing stepping out of right/wrong thinking and into exploring.

> As teachers develop their skills, they naturally develop an "ear" for the kinds of areas that are important to highlight and investigate within the teaching process. Certain themes are prominent at different phases in the course. In the preparation for each class it is important that these are brought to mind, and then in the actuality of the teaching the immediacy of participants' experience is given priority, and linked to these themes as they naturally emerge.

Jane's experiments with noticing experiences more intentionally in everyday life had offered her an encouraging glimpse of the potential of mindfulness. She was enjoying small moments of being at ease in a new way. The formal practices challenged her more strongly, however, because they put her into direct contact with the urge to escape or avoid that she used to protect herself from aversive experience. At the end of the session, the teacher checked in with her individually and encouraged her to make contact during the week if she was struggling.

Jane was feeling challenged by the learning process but at the same time she was curious and willing to stay with the exploration. Although she had suffered from recurrent depression and suicidality for many years and it had dominated how she lived her life between episodes, she had never systematically investigated the particular nature of the vulnerability. The themes that were emerging in her own process, and in the group as a whole, struck a vivid chord with her.

Session 3: Gathering the Scattered Mind

Jane found that she could engage more easily with the mindful movement practice. Challenging though it was, the body scan had introduced her to the theme of bringing attention to the specifics of raw sensory experience. It then became feasible for her to translate this learning into feeling sensations in the body as it moves. Later, this became an important gateway into mindfulness at times when she felt agitated and when it seemed impossible to sit still to practice.

She found that her experience resonated with one of the other participants, Penny, who shared her experiences after the first Session 3 practice (mindful movement):

> PENNY: I found it easier to concentrate on the stretches than I did on the body scan
>
> TEACHER: What did you notice? What caught your attention?

The teacher is supporting Penny to anchor her descriptions of experience in specific "noticings."

> PENNY: I felt totally here. My mind wasn't wandering away because I was moving. I was concentrating on what it felt like, but with the body scan I can really sort of go off.
>
> TEACHER: So something about moving. What difference did that make to the sensation of moving, do you think? Can you pinpoint?

Again the teacher brings Penny back to specific tangible sensations.

> PENNY: I think it just made the sensations clearer so that I was more aware of them today whereas before I had to really make myself think about each toe and everything. And today I didn't have to make myself do it.
>
> TEACHER: Ah, so the sensation of movement gave your mind a clearer point of focus.

The teacher is staying in connection with Penny and with her experience as she supports her to "unfold" the memory of her experience.

> PENNY: Yes I felt comfortable with it but not very flexible—I found that I couldn't do all the movements—my knees were hurting.

Note how Penny started with a fairly neutral area for exploration and has now moved to a difficult aspect. The sense of safely builds through the connection within the inquiry, and the process reconnects participants to the specifics of their experience. The inquiry then moved to exploring the process of working with physical boundaries in the practice, how these interfaced with ideas about how the body could or should be, and the emotions that arose around these struggles.

Moving back to Jane's experience during the week of practice, she had discovered that there were moments in which she could notice difficult aspects of experience (particularly discrepancy-based "things should be different" thoughts), attend to them briefly, and then redirect attention to body sensations. During the home practice review she shared some of the challenge and doubt that she was experiencing. The heightened level of noticing was bringing some pleasure—she had never previously taken time to savor her life, and during the week had enjoyed sitting in her conservatory (which backed onto open countryside) and looking out over the view. Similarly, her granddaughter was immensely dear to her and she was discovering a new pleasure in spending time with her without an agenda. Alongside this, though, she had felt uncharacteristically tearful and had experienced strong waves of anxiety. She was unnerved by this because once again it left her feeling out of control and fearful that these experiences could escalate and her mood could descend. She had contacted the teacher during the week to talk over her concerns and fears. The teacher had spent time exploring and acknowledging her experience. For Jane, the sense of threat that unpleasant thoughts and emotions roused was immense because they were so strongly associated with her most despairing times. Together with the teacher, she investigated further the theme of working at the edge of what was possible for her—it was helpful that this had subsequently arisen in the session in relation to working with physical boundaries in the body. The teacher explored with Jane how she could stay with the meditation practices, but modulate the intensity of exposure to her thinking mind in various ways.

> When the fear of entrapment is strong, it is particularly important for participants to know that they are in "the driver's seat" when it comes to making choices about how to engage with the meditation practices.

Detailed conversations on how to modulate the practice in ways that are responsive to a participant's particular boundaries are sometimes easier to have outside the group context. There is a delicate balance between encouraging participants to stay with the discipline of the practices *and* supporting them to work flexibly with them. Specifically, from conversations after the class, it emerged that Jane found that the "sense door" of *seeing* anchored her in the present moment, so she found it helpful to know that it was perfectly okay to work with opening her eyes during the practice. It also became clear that the shorter sitting meditation practices and the mindful movement practices felt more accessible, so she decided to prioritize these. Finally, she found the experience of bringing her attention into her body as she moved very workable, so she decided to allow more time for the walk to work. Alongside this she planned to continue with the longer formal "physically still" practices that she found particularly challenging, but to know that she could take care of herself by stepping back and shifting to a practice that in the moment felt accessible. During the class the teacher and Jane arranged that she could choose, during any of the guided practices, to move out of the group and sit in a chair by the window, and so make a transition to a seeing practice. The fear of entrapment was strong, so it was particularly important for Jane to know that she was in "the driver's seat" when it came to making choices about how to engage with the practices.

Session 4: Recognizing Aversion

The theme of working with reactivity and aversion was at the heart of the exploration in this session. The 40-minute sitting meditation was introduced for the first time at the beginning of the session—a practice which on this occasion included the noise of builder's machinery outside—and then the teacher opened the inquiry.

> "So let's take some time to reflect back on this practice, and really inviting you as we move into this talking time to stay very close to your immediate experience. So this is like another meditation practice, developing the skill to track your experience, to notice how you are moment by moment. So whether you are talking or listening, just being open to how things are for you. So—how was this practice? What did you notice?"

Notice how the teacher is inviting the group to begin to apply their mindfulness skills in other aspects of their lives—here to the process of talking and sharing. Participants are invited to experiment with bringing mindfulness into the fabric of their days in a variety of ways, and this is embodied by encouraging continuity of kindly attention throughout the class. Let's leave Jane for a moment and see how another participant, Suzi, shared experience of her struggle with the sounds of workmen outside the room:

> SUZI: I was totally wound up by that noise outside—every time it came on I was like "Oh, for goodness sake."
>
> TEACHER: Yeah.
>
> SUZI: And then the noise would stop and I would swing into nearly falling asleep, and then the noise would come again and I would think "oh for goodness sake," and I just couldn't relax.
>
> TEACHER: So when the sound came on there was this immediate thought—this sense of really not wanting this.
>
> SUZI: Yes, yes.
>
> TEACHER: And did you notice how that was showing up in the body?

The teacher is inviting meta-awareness of experience—from a participant-observer stance, seeing the different elements of experience and how they interact (i.e., being simultaneously inside the experience and being able to see it for what it is).

> SUZI: Yeah, I got this feeling of like nerves you know like butterflies and I'm thinking "This is really annoying me," and I've got to concentrate and I'm getting more wound up 'cause I can't concentrate 'cause of that noise . . . and then it would stop and then it would start again and I'd start getting wound up again and the butterflies would come again.

Notice that Suzi starts by describing some experiences in her body but reverts to the more familiar territory of describing thoughts. The teacher encourages her to ground her noticing of sensations in specifics.

> TEACHER: So where were the butterflies?
>
> SUZI: Sort of here. (*gesturing to her abdominal area*)

TEACHER: Here (*mirroring gesture*)—so could you say a little bit about the feeling?

SUZI: It felt like something is moving about in there—sounds gross. (*laughing*)

TEACHER: Moving about . . .

SUZI: Yes—like this bubbling blupping sort of feeling.

TEACHER: Yes—and then the sound would stop and what would happen to this. (*hand on abdomen*)

SUZI: It would go—but then I would find myself waiting for the sound to come back.

TEACHER: Okay, and what was happening during the waiting—was it thinking "When is this going to start up again?" or was it more a feeling in your body?

SUZI: It was definitely thinking—"It's going to start up again and I'm trying to relax here."

TEACHER: So you were more aware of thoughts than of your body?

SUZI: Oh, yes.

TEACHER: And there was something interesting that you said, Suzi—so the sounds started up, the thoughts came about the sounds and then there was this, (*hand on abdomen*) and then there was other thoughts like "and I'm trying to relax." What effect did these extra thoughts have?

SUZI: They wound me up more—I was trying too hard to relax—instead noticing my experience I found myself concentrating more on what was going on outside.

TEACHER: Ah—so you said something very important there—"I was trying too hard to relax." Isn't it extraordinary to see how these extra thoughts creep in to influence us? (*looking around the group and then back to Suzi*)

SUZI: It is—I was trying to relax, and I was listening to the thoughts more than I was listening to the practice, and they stopped me from relaxing. (*laughing*)

Notice that rather than moving straight into a "teaching point," the teacher gives space to Suzi to make her own discovery—to recognize for herself how these thoughts and the way she gave attention to them influenced her. The teacher then reframes the learning for the whole group:

> TEACHER: Yes—and your attention was more with these thoughts so you were less in touch with the feel of things in your body. (*turning to the group*) So this is what happens when we have a goal. So we are sitting here, (*miming sitting in meditation*) we are setting out and there is this plan we have "I'm going to get relaxed" and then the sound outside starts up—and it's getting in the way of getting to our goal of getting relaxed. So there's this sense of I'm here (*pointing to where she is sitting*) and I need to be there (*pointing to the other side of the room*) and this thing is getting in the way. Does this connect to what you experienced here? (*turning back to Suzi*)
>
> SUZI: Yes—it really does—I can see how my thoughts are running the show. (*laughing–group laughter*)
>
> TEACHER: Did anyone else find that this pattern of wanting things to be a certain way showed up in the practice?

The inquiry then opened into other participants sharing a range of experiences that were difficult. Jane shared her own experience of struggling with "I can't do this" and "I should be able to do this" sort of thoughts. It was tremendously helpful for her to see that the same pattern of internal reactivity crops up whether the unwanted experience is initially outside (e.g., a sound, an annoying event at work), or a thought (e.g., "I can't do this"). Through this, she was beginning to really notice, with some interest—and perhaps even a little compassion—her familiar reactive patterns of fighting her way through life and being fierce with herself.

Session 5: Allowing and Letting Be

The theme of "doing battle" with experience was prominent in Session 5 also. Jane and the teacher had this exchange after the first sitting meditation (within which there was an invitation to turn the attention toward a difficult experience and explore thoughts, sensations, and emotions around this experience).

JANE: I really struggled. I was holding myself tight. It got to the stage where my hand was numb.

TEACHER: Ahhh—so it was really difficult—would you mind saying some more?

JANE: My mind was wandering constantly. I'm not in a good place today anyway. My mind is just constantly going. When you say concentrate on your breathing my mind is just like all over the place. And when you say relax—my mind is thinking these horrible things.

Notice that Jane has interpreted the guidance to keep coming back to the breath as an injunction to "concentrate on it" and has an idea that she should relax—even though these were not part of the guidance. This illustrates the habitual tendency to create goals about how things should be and what needs to be achieved.

TEACHER: So in *this* practice you experienced a lot of challenging thoughts?

JANE: Yes—really horrible thoughts about how I can't do this now, and memories from the past coming back to the surface—stuff I don't want to think about.

TEACHER: Ah—so how did you work with this just now in this practice?

Jane was vulnerable as she was speaking—there was both a wobble and an angry force behind her voice. The teacher moved forward in her chair, gave space through pauses and silence and stayed with supporting the unfolding of the exploration.

JANE: (*gesturing–tight clenched fists, tension in face*)

TEACHER: And were there emotions that came along with this? (*mirroring Jane's gestures*)

JANE: I just feel so angry at how much pain my mind causes and I want to get on top of it. I get really angry because I want to do this but I can't. I can't stop my mind thinking.

TEACHER: Yes, yes—it is so understandable that you want this—I think each one of us here can relate to what you are saying.

The teacher pauses and looks around class. Again the group is important in underlining the universality of the human yearning for a peaceful mind, and the frustration felt when this cannot be brought about by an act of will.

JANE: I want to have a nice time in my life but it is like I have the angel and the devil living inside me and they are always arguing and I say to them "Shut up, you can talk later."

TEACHER: So it's like a battle—Jane versus mind.

JANE: Yes, I am fighting with my mind to get back into the present moment and pushing to listen to you. I am telling myself "just concentrate on what you are saying" and then I think "ooh, I've missed that part" and then I can't let go of having not done it right.

TEACHER: So your thoughts are ordering you about and being critical of you, you are trying to ignore them, push them away, and "do" the practice; there is a lot of frustration and anger; and you feel really tight in your body.

JANE: Yes—big time.

TEACHER: And understandably you don't want any of this.

JANE: No, I don't!

TEACHER: How did the battle play out for you in this practice as we went along?

JANE: It just got stronger and stronger.

TEACHER: So you got kind of locked into the battle?

JANE: Yes and then I opted out—I just sat here and kept my mind busy thinking about work.

TEACHER: Ah—so this is really interesting to notice—I wonder if this is familiar—this moving between being in a battle with the mind and then trying to get away from it by distracting?

JANE: Yes—that's what I do. (*laughing*)

TEACHER: Is this familiar to others? (*looking around the group*)— this getting locked into battle, then trying to get away. (*murmurs and smiles from group–sense of recognition*)

The teacher affirmed battling as a strategy that works for Jane in many spheres of her life—she is a "get-up-and-go" sort of person, it helps her to achieve practical tasks. The problem emerges when she tries to deal with her unwanted thoughts and emotions using this same approach. The exploration focuses on how it might be possible to relate to painful thoughts and images (including of suicide) in a way that allows them to remain in experience, without resorting to an escape mode of mind that then leads to "arrested flight" when it doesn't work (see Chapter 2). It is tremendously important to acknowledge the immense painfulness, sense of urgency, and accompanying feelings of loss of control and being overwhelmed when such mental pain arrives.

The teacher then reminded the group about the possibility that the practice invites us to experiment with—the possibility of neither engaging with the thoughts (by arguing or ruminating), nor trying to get away from them (by distraction or suppression), but instead seeing them simply as thoughts arising and passing within the mind, and repeatedly bringing the attention to rest on sensations in the body. She then turned back to Jane to explore how this might practically be done. The underpinning intention is to explore ways of "gently being with" painful experience so that it gradually becomes workable.

TEACHER: So in this practice, when you were in this battle with your thoughts, and you were feeling angry—could you say what is the feeling in your body?

JANE: Like this (*clenching fists*)

TEACHER: And how does this feel? (*mirroring fists*)

JANE: I can feel my nails in the palm of my hand and tightness up here (*signaling up her arms*)—and my face is tight.

TEACHER: Ah—so how does this feel? (*gesturing around the face*)

JANE: Hard . . . and (*pausing to notice*) a bit trembly too.

TEACHER: Hard and trembly—anything else?

JANE: My jaw is aching—I didn't notice that before.

TEACHER: Yes—it is interesting to notice that there are a lot of feelings in the body that we aren't usually tuned into. So there is hands, arms, face, and in other parts of your body? (*gesturing around the body*)

JANE: Ummm (*pausing*) I can feel now how I am holding myself—like I am trying to push myself up out of the chair.

TEACHER: Ah yes—(*turning to the group*) so maybe we could all notice the feel of the body here on the chair—is there holding, tightness, or maybe some softness . . . (*pausing to give space to this mini-practice, then turning back to Jane*) What do you notice as you stay with the feeling of your body with the chair?

JANE: I can see that the tightness goes right down to my feet . . . (*laughing*)

TEACHER: So this is really good noticing—so this is what the practice is inviting us to do—to notice thoughts but then to leave them be and step into feeling things in the body.

JANE: Yes.

TEACHER: There will be this dance between getting caught up in thoughts and then coming back. There's always this possibility of coming back—even if it's just feeling the breath for a moment and then getting caught up—and actually for this not to be a battle—just keeping it simple. Not simple in the sense that it is easy, but simple in the sense that coming back doesn't need to be a battle.

The teacher connected this exploration with the theme introduced in the sitting meditation at the beginning of the session. Up until now the invitation has consistently been to notice other aspects of experience as they occur, but then to bring the mind back to a specific focus on sensation. Now the additional possibility is offered of deliberately allowing difficulty to be center stage and giving time to explore it. The teacher pointed out how this sense of "battling" could itself be a good example of a difficulty which could be worked with in practice by noticing the play of thoughts and emotions, and then deliberately turning the attention toward the feelings of tightness, tension, and holding in the body—and bringing the breath to these places as a way to support exploration.

The possibility that the practice invites may need coming back to again and again in the class, in one way or another. What is this possibility? To explore the middle way of neither engaging with the thoughts (by arguing or ruminating), on the one hand, nor trying to get away from them (by distraction or suppression), on the other. Instead the invitation is to see them simply as thoughts arising and passing within the mind. How is this done? By repeatedly bringing the attention to rest on sensations in the body.

Interestingly, later in the session during the home practice review, Jane shared her experience of the flip side of trying to get rid of unwanted experience—trying to pursue wanted experience:

JANE: When it does go well I do enjoy it—there have been moments when I have felt easy in the practice and it's a nice feeling—I want to feel like that again.

TEACHER: Again I think that what you are saying is something that we all can relate to (*looking around–nods from group–affirming the naturalness of this pattern*) . . . so great for all of us to enjoy and rest into these moments when they come—but we are not chasing nice feelings here. We're learning that whatever happens, it's okay, it is workable, and doing that moment by moment by moment—so if anger is here, anger is here . . . if ease is here, ease is here.

This is often a challenging phase in the program as participants are still in the early stages of developing their mindfulness skills, and are already exploring the relevance of this learning to the most difficult of experiences. Later in this session the group investigated the patterns of thoughts, sensations, and emotions that arise at deeply challenging times when low mood and suicidal thoughts and feelings are present. Jane was tremendously challenged by this process, but at the same time was struck by the similarity in reactive patterns to these difficult times that emerged in the group.

For the teacher too, it is challenging work. It is not possible to teach this without connecting to the vulnerability that is inherent in all of us. We would often find that during this phase in the program we were more sensitive and vulnerable in our wider life. So long as we were willing and open to work with this vulnerability in our lives and in how we were teaching, we found that it supported the process— strengthened our levels of courage and confidence while we were teaching. While it is clear that the teacher has primary responsibility for creating the culture within the class, we found that the teaching felt more fluent and effective when we had a broader trust that participants' learning is not dependent on the teacher being completely perfect, but rather on how vulnerability and imperfections are held within the process.

Session 6: Thoughts Are Not Facts

The theme of this session was at the heart of what Jane most struggled with in her learning process. Initially she had thought that the meditation practices actually increased the volume of her thoughts, but she was recognizing now that a continual stream of thinking was always present, and that, beyond her awareness, it was influencing her wider experience. Indeed, she could see now how much energy she habitually put into keeping thoughts at bay, and was becoming more aware of the particular strategies she used and what was driving them. But it was painful and challenging to look at and work with these tendencies. As she experimented with allowing thoughts to enter her mind, she was strongly aware of their painful emotional impact. It was challenging to stay present with the waves of sensation she experienced in her trunk and with the ripples of tightness through her body. Nonetheless, it gave her a place to anchor her attention each time she got swept away into trains of thought and was gradually becoming more natural. She was learning that by repeatedly redirecting her attention to her bodily experience, she was breaking a cycle of reactivity, and by so doing ceasing to feed the perpetuation of negative cycles.

In the inquiry following the first practice Jane and the teacher had this interaction:

JANE: There are some thoughts that I have that I can naturally just dismiss, but others I can't do that. Some thoughts I get stuck with—and it can be for days and days.

TEACHER: Right, yes—so this is important to notice—some thoughts are easier to acknowledge and let be and other thoughts are much more sticky—we get entangled in them. And, as we've been exploring over these last weeks, these difficult thoughts have a strong influence on how we feel—emotionally and physically—and on what we do. What did you notice about these sticky thoughts in this practice?

Notice how the teacher reframes Jane's "dismiss" into "acknowledge and let be." The inquiry process does offer opportunities for subtly supporting participants to shift to a gentler, more compassionate mode of relating to experience. The teacher responds in a general way, highlighting this theme, but then focuses the inquiry on exploration of a specific example of this phenomenon.

> JANE: I had this sudden thought that when I sent a difficult e-mail today to one of my team that I had clicked "reply all" rather than just "reply" to her, and that what I said would be right through the whole team now.
>
> TEACHER: And how did this thought affect you?
>
> JANE: It started me up on loads of thoughts—"How could I be so stupid," "What will everyone think of me," "How will I undo the damage I have caused." Of course I don't even know if it's true—I'll check when I go home.

The scenario that Jane had imagined connected her with emotional memories of episodes when she perceived that she had failed and so brought back "online" feelings of shame and guilt that were associated with these past times.

> TEACHER: Yes, interesting to notice that whether or not they are true, in the moment of thinking these thoughts they have a strong effect. So cascades of thoughts were triggered by this idea that you might have made a mistake. Did you notice how your body was feeling?
>
> JANE: Well, I did but I couldn't keep my mind there—I kept pinging back to thinking.
>
> TEACHER: Yes—this is very natural—so what did you notice when you did bring your attention to your body?

The teacher emphasizes the naturalness of the wandering mind—a reminder that it is not a mistake that it wanders.

JANE: Feeling sick, heart beating, I was jumpy—I wanted to leave and go and check it out.

TEACHER: So your attention was jumping between these thoughts, then noticing sensations in your body and the impulse to move?

JANE: Yes—I guess.

TEACHER: Do you have a sense what difference it made, even coming away for a moment to feel your body?

JANE: Well, it was different—in the past I wouldn't have stayed here—I would have left the room—at least I'm still sitting here talking about it. (*laughing*)

TEACHER: Ah, so this is big—you have discovered that you don't need to act on your thoughts immediately!

JANE: Yes—and my thoughts didn't get as extreme as they often do.

TEACHER: Say more.

JANE: Well, that sort of thought can often quickly lead into really horrible stuff.

TEACHER: Critical, judgmental thoughts?

JANE: Yes—attacking myself—there was a bit of that but not so much as usual and I didn't take it quite so seriously.

TEACHER: (*turning to the whole group*) So important for us to notice that each time we do bring attention to the body we have interrupted the thinking mind—it might start up again, but in that moment, there is a pause . . . and also this possibility that Jane has noticed of horrible thoughts being present but not taking them as the truth.

> You cannot plan what you will think, nor can you stop thoughts you do not want, but you can influence how you relate to them by redirecting your attention to sensations in the body and bringing gentle kindness to yourself in these moments.

Jane was thus beginning to learn how to relate to her thoughts in ways that did not feed them. This is not easy, and infusing the whole teaching with compassion is an important part of the process. It is kindness for oneself that enables one to ride these difficult painful times when cascades of toxic thoughts are pouring through. Much of this is communicated implicitly by the teacher through his or her embodiment of the practice and the atmosphere that this creates in the class. This compassionate atmosphere is very different from the internal atmosphere of participants' minds, and it points toward a possibility that can gradually begin to grow. You cannot plan what you will think, nor can you stop thoughts you do not want, but you can influence how you are with them by redirecting attention to sensations in the body and bringing gentle kindness to yourself in these moments.

Session 7: How Can I Best Take Care of Myself?

Jane had been exploring from the beginning of the course how she could bring her mindfulness skills into everyday life. Over the last 2 weeks since the exploration of patterns of avoidance in Session 5, she had been deliberately noticing reactive behavioral patterns. She had in general withdrawn from contact with friends over the years, but in the last week had consciously chosen to say "yes" to an invitation to meet up with some old school friends for a drink—"I've put my head in the sand for so many years—I want to do it different now and try out new things." She was able to recognize how this decision asked her to turn toward challenging emotions, thoughts, and sensations (she felt nervous and had thoughts about what they might be thinking about her), but was able to use her mindfulness skills to ride these. The more explicit investigation in this session on daily activity and the potential for mindfully influencing choices extended her sense of possibility in this area.

Jane's greatest risk factor for a future episode of depression was becoming burnt out and exhausted because of overworking and putting too much pressure on herself. The main drivers to her pattern of pushing to continually be doing and achieving were the attempt to keep a distance from her thoughts, to keep up with the high standards she set for herself, and the automatic habitual nature of this pattern (see Chapter 2 and the discussion of how perfectionism makes some people more sensitive to anything that might be construed as failure). Mindfulness practice had helped her to understand and recognize these drivers, and to step out of automatic habit patterns more often. She was at an early stage in learning how to use these recognitions to support taking skillful action. Significantly, though, she had now become curious, actively willing to experiment, and interested in noticing how her choices relating to activity influenced things both externally and internally.

She was particularly struck by how variable her experience was—"Last week one day I felt really anxious, the next day I felt really calm, another day I had a headache and was feeling tired." In the past she had held the same standards for herself whatever she was feeling. Her mood could cascade down at moments when her impatience with tiredness led to irritability, which led to reactive behaviors, which led to streams of critical thoughts and related emotions. She was now recognizing the importance of taking her own "internal weather" into account. During the work on developing a relapse prevention action plan, she was able to fine-tune how to recognize these shifts so as to be better equipped to tailor her responses to them.

Session 8: Maintaining and Extending the New Learning

In the second half of the final session, time was given to developing the relapse plans further. Following work in small groups, each participant was invited to share one thing that "feels particularly important for you at these difficult times." The responses showed that mindfulness skills were influencing behavioral choices and responses to aspects of internal experience—how participants were relating to thoughts, sensations, and emotions. Here are some of them from the group:

> "I need to get enough sleep because when I get really exhausted my mood is more likely to slip . . . but also to go gently with myself when I am tired."
> "I need to put less pressure on myself."
> "It is important for me to make sure I eat regularly."
> "Give myself more spaces in the day to pause."
> "I'm working with being more accepting of myself. I can't change me so best accept myself as I am and be okay with who I am as I am."

"I want to notice how I pull away from contact with people when I am feeling low and to see if I can stay in contact."

"To spend more time doing the things I love—particularly being in my garden."

"To remind myself that looking after myself isn't selfish, it is essential."

The exploration around how best to stay in touch with what is important was of key importance for Jane. She continued to struggle to engage with the longer sitting meditations, but had a range of practices that did feel possible for her. The teacher encouraged the group to settle into a form of practice that felt sustainable over the next 4 weeks until the follow-up session. Jane had some trepidation about the end of the class because her learning felt new, and she recognized that the pull back into reactive patterns was strong. The teacher emphasized that this was just the beginning of the exploration. The key was to develop a regular discipline (a word that comes from the Latin *discipulus,* which means *student* and does not mean *being hard on oneself*). So future practice was about "being a student," investigating the implementation of practice in everyday life, so that the connection with the learning is kept alive. Within this it was important to make this her own, and be open to how the learning unfolds. In the closing round Jane shared an observation about what had happened during the previous week when she had felt low for a couple of days. It struck a chord with the group and, although it may not seem much, for Jane, it represented a major step forward in her journey to look after herself when low mood threatens to overwhelm her. This was her comment: "I had low mood, low mood didn't have me."

Jane came to the two follow-up sessions (at 1 month and 6 months following the end of the program). She continued to be actively engaged with exploring the interface between mindfulness skills and her experience. She had had some difficult times when her mood had dipped. Significantly, though, rather than trying to push through these times, she had eased up and deliberately taken more care of herself. This felt counterintuitive to her. It seemed strange that *allowing herself to be more vulnerable seemed to make her less vulnerable.*

The question that this chapter is addressing is "How does MBCT enable transformation?" Jane's journey through the program illustrates that the shifts that participants make are often quite subtle but have a radical effect. A seemingly small shift in orientation and perspective can have a profound impact on patterns of behavior and on ways of relating to experience.

Concluding Remarks

From an MBCT teacher's perspective, this is also difficult work. Teachers are holding some challenging tensions within the learning process. On the one hand, they must offer their participants the program as intended, respecting its current evidence base. On the other hand, they must also be sensitively attentive to the immediate responses and needs of these particular participants, at this particular moment. They will also need to be aware of their own inevitable reactions, especially to difficult times, and choose wisely how best to respond to these. Thus leading an 8-week course (especially with people at risk of suicidal depression) is a demanding process, requiring high levels of mindful awareness, empathy, embedded theoretical knowledge of the two traditions (ancient contemplative practices and modern scientific) on which MBCT draws, and clinical skill.

Within this context, what does it mean to be competent? How can we know that we are carrying out the program as intended, and to the high standard deserved by our participants? This question recurred throughout our work on the trial and within our ongoing work of training others to teach MBCT. The two chapters in Part III focus specifically on this area first by exploring the question: "How do we recognize skillful teaching when we see it?", then by addressing the issues from the internal perspective of the teacher within the teaching process.

PART III

TRAINING TEACHERS AND DEFINING COMPETENCE

CHAPTER 16

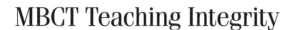

MBCT Teaching Integrity

Assessing Mindfulness-Based Teaching Skills

A large part of the responsibility for the learning process within MBCT lies with the participant. Choosing to take an MBCT class involves an investment of time and a willingness to engage with an often personally challenging learning process. The depth and extent of participants' learning is thus strongly influenced by the depth and extent to which they are able to commit to and engage with the program. This is influenced by factors within participants and by their life circumstances at the time. Additionally, right from the preclass interview, the class teacher plays a significant role in acting as a catalyst for engagement.

Over the years of developing mindfulness-based interventions (MBIs), including both Kabat-Zinn's MBSR and the later adaptation of this in MBCT, considerable thought and care has been given to how the learning environment can offer optimum conditions for participants to make this (often difficult) leap to engage and then stay with the learning process. The question of what good mindfulness-based teaching looks like, and what training programs need to offer to enable trainees to develop core skills, has been a matter of considerable debate and discussion. These are difficult questions, because the work of being a mindfulness-based teacher is tremendously personal.

The teaching is based on the premise that participants' movement into mindful connection with direct experience is largely facilitated by the teachers' capacity to engage with experience in just this way. This is intimate, interior work, and hence it can seem reductionist and disrespectful to attempt to operationalize it in any way. And yet, these questions ask for responses that are as clear as possible. The approach can only be effectively developed and disseminated if there is clarity about what particular teaching skills are required and how they are developed.

When Zindel Segal, Mark Williams, and John Teasdale were piloting an early version of MBCT during the development of the approach, they describe their default tendency to revert back into the familiar territory of cognitive-behavioral therapy (CBT) (see Chapter 3; Segal et al., 2013, pp. 45–59). As participants moved into exploration of difficulty, Segal, Williams, and Teasdale would sometimes lose confidence in the mindfulness model and be tempted to take refuge in the CBT concepts and treatment methods that they had previously learned and become familiar with, and whose effectiveness they had experienced. Over the years, in our mindfulness-based teacher training work, we have seen a similar phenomenon repeatedly playing out. Whatever the nature of the training engaged in before learning to become an MBCT/MBSR teacher, there is a tendency to revert to this familiar territory during teaching practice, especially when the going gets tough. This reversion might be to another therapeutic orientation, or to another form of meditation practice the learner is familiar with. The importance of staying true to the model and to the practices being learned and practiced has become increasingly clear to us. When at pivotal moments or times of difficulty the teacher loses confidence and crosses over into other models and practices, the opportunity to support participants in deepening their own confidence in the approach is lost, at the very moment when it is most needed. The practice of MBCT and the model underpinning it have been rigorously evaluated through repeated cycles of theoretical development and empirical testing. This is not a question of saying that it is "better" than other models or practices, but rather that the potency of any model relies on adherence to its core ingredients—in short, teaching integrity.

In this chapter, we describe work led by Rebecca Crane and conducted at the mindfulness centers at Bangor, Exeter, and Oxford Universities. This work ran in parallel with the research described in this book, and its intention was to articulate the core characteristics of mindfulness-based teaching integrity and to develop a methodology for assessing it. The result was the "Mindfulness-Based Interventions: Teaching Assessment Criteria" (MBI:TAC; Crane, Soulsby, et al., 2012) which is freely accessible online (*http://mindfulnessteachersuk.org. uk/pdf/MBI-TACJune2012.pdf*). We also describe how it was for us to attempt something many people consider to be by definition impossible: to create a tool capable of defining and assessing the integrity and quality of mindfulness-based teaching.

It is important to be clear, before we embark upon detailed discussion of how we developed our procedures, that the intention was not to produce an assessment tool exclusive to MBCT, but rather a means of evaluating the integrity of all mindfulness-based programs that, like MBCT, are based on the core MBSR structure and teaching process. Certainly, elements of MBCT spring directly from its psychological (and in particular cognitive) roots, for example, the focus on depressive and despairing cognitions that we have described in the chapters in Part II. However, MBCT also shares much of its curriculum with MBSR, from which it developed. Not only that, but the style of the teaching and the experiential learning process are held in common, as will be clear from those aspects of the MBI:TAC which we have included in this chapter. So, although MBCT will be our prime focus in this chapter because it is the approach we used with our vulnerable participants, readers whose teaching and training practice draws on other mindfulness-based interventions will nonetheless find the discussion directly relevant to what they do.

What Is Intervention Integrity?

"Intervention integrity" is the term used to describe the degree to which an intervention is implemented as intended. Broadly, the concept has three dimensions: adherence, differentiation, and competence.

- "Adherence" refers to the extent to which the teacher/therapist applies the appropriate "ingredients" at the appropriate time points, and refrains from introducing methods and curriculum elements that are not recognized as part of the approach.
- "Differentiation" refers to the degree to which the approach can be distinguished from other approaches.
- "Competence" is a more complex dimension, and refers to the teacher's skill in delivering the intervention.

Why is it important to consider the question of MBCT teaching integrity? Verification of the integrity of an approach is important for a number of reasons:

- In MBCT research trials, delivering the teaching as intended and to a sufficiently high quality is a key variable in interpreting the results, and may well influence outcome for participants. In order to be sure of this, systems need to be built into research trial governance to assess levels of adherence, differentiation, and competence.
- These issues are not confined to research trial contexts. In training contexts too there needs to be clarity regarding the particular skills that are being developed, and systems to ensure that the training is effective in achieving its aims.
- In the context of university validated postgraduate MBCT teacher training programs (such as those offered at the United Kingdom universities of Bangor, Oxford, and Exeter), formal assessment of teaching practice is required for the award of academic credits. For this purpose, assessment criteria and the assessment process must be entirely clear and transparent.
- Systems to check teaching integrity are also an important ingredient in successful implementation. MBCT is increasingly being commissioned and implemented in the United Kingdom National Health Service and other settings. There is a risk that, in the drive to implement a promising approach, the very factors that give rise to its promise are lost through a dilution of its integrity as it is rolled out. Nationally agreed-upon benchmarks and governance assessing readiness to teach help to ensure that slippage from the core model does not take

place during the transition from research to practice (Rycroft-Malone et al., 2014).

• Teachers also have a clinical and ethical responsibility for ensuring that programs are delivered to a high level of integrity and in line with available evidence. Supervision plays a key role in supporting this and many are now using the MBI:TAC as a reflective tool within this context (Evans, Crane et al., 2014).

We thus found that, within various areas of our work, the challenging question of how to work skillfully with teaching integrity kept recurring. How could we reliably and validly assess students' teaching skills within our master's programs? How could we assess the integrity of teaching within classes conducted as part of research projects? How could the issue of teaching integrity be addressed in developing guidance for implementing MBCT within health care services? In 2009 we took the step of turning more systematically to this issue. The Bangor, Exeter, and Oxford teams came together to delve more deeply into the question of how best to articulate the breadth and depth of mindfulness-based teaching, and how to use this as a basis for developing an assessment tool.

We started by pooling experiences that had emerged at our respective centers on the theme of competency. Interestingly, in the early assessment work that we conducted within our master's programs using checklists of domains of mindfulness-based teaching, we discovered that our double marking (two trainers independently grading a piece of teaching) was highly reliable—certainly as good as we achieved when marking academic assignments using well-established criteria. So it was clear that there were consistent aspects to the teaching process which our training teams could recognize. However, at this point in time, we were less skilled at describing in words what we recognized. Specific and explicit aspects of the teaching were relatively amenable to description, but other aspects were harder to describe. When our trainers were pressed to put words to these less definable aspects, they would say things like: "The appropriate elements within the session were all there, and the teacher had a warm and pleasant manner, but it all left me feeling a bit flat and uninspired"; or "There was something in the atmosphere that seemed to really invited the group to come alongside the teacher and investigate." The challenge we faced was to develop an assessment tool that accounted for the multiple processes that are simultaneously in action in a mindfulness-based class, including those sometimes defined as indefinable.

Developing the MBI:TAC

Although mindfulness-based teaching pedagogy places a strong emphasis on the teachers' implicit understandings and personal mindfulness practice, it is clear that this must be communicated within the teaching if it is to have any influence. We therefore became interested in recognizing and describing how this inner work becomes visible, audible, and felt through the behavior of the teacher. Our intention was to develop an assessment tool that would describe what is seen, heard, and sensed when participating in skillful teaching. We aimed to operationalize teaching integrity by focusing both on assessors' observations *and* on their direct experience of the teaching itself. Observation and experience are thus focused on what assessors see (behavior, nonverbal communication), what they feel (visceral), what they hear (language), and how these "data" combine to become the overall experience of the teaching.

The development of the MBI:TAC thus involved close analysis of mindfulness-based teaching by a group of teacher trainers from mindfulness centers at the Universities of Bangor, Exeter, and Oxford. In a series of meetings over a period of 18 months, we met to watch audiovisual recordings of teaching sessions and assessed them using the tool we were developing. We had detailed and often passionate discussions, as we teased out the subtleties of the teaching process and the language we were using to describe it. Between meetings we tried out the tool to assess teaching in our respective centers and shared experiences by e-mail and phone conference calls. We searched for personal and consensual meaning as we built domain titles, descriptors, and competency levels. Over time, through these influences, we made changes and amendments to the tool—adjusting the number of domains and competence levels, and refining the language we used to increase specificity.

This development and pilot phase was framed within an inquiry process that was open to the felt sense, felt meanings, and subtleties of the teaching process before ideas formed as clearly defined and recognizable constructs. We were under no illusion about the difficulty of creating a tool that claims to "assess" what really happens in mindfulness-based teaching. We recognized that the work we were engaged in was part of an endeavor to bridge the paradigms that each one of us on the development team inhabited: on the one hand, the investigation paradigm of Western scientific methodology, with a focus on measurement, outcome, and evaluation; and, on the other hand, the mindfulness-based paradigm of nonstriving, letting be, and engagement with process in the moment. There were tensions inherent in this process. We had to deal with our own doubts, and with our fears about the skepticism of mindfulness teacher colleagues around the world. We found ourselves wanting to reassure them that the tool we were developing was not simply a "tick box" list of how to "do" mindfulness-based teaching, or a reductionist approach to a complex process. We also wanted to develop a methodology that was robust—that did indeed enable experienced trainers reliably and validly to assess teaching integrity. As we embarked on the journey, we did not know where it would take us, or whether the endeavor was indeed possible. Would we be able to develop a tool that was practical and usable in training and research contexts, that accurately assessed the construct of mindfulness-based teaching integrity, and that could reliably be used by assessors? Is it possible to quantify how well a teacher is doing in delivering a mindfulness-based course? Can relational qualities such as warmth and connection be assessed? What about embodied and experientially felt qualities, such as nonstriving and present-moment focus? As best we could, we brought to the process an open-minded curiosity as to where this journey would take us.

Refining the MBI:TAC

Developing the criteria took about 18 months, by which time we had created a working version of the MBI:TAC. We then implemented it within our three postgraduate mindfulness-based teacher training programs, conducting research on its reliability and validity when used in this context (see Research section below). Like the warp and the weft of a piece of woven cloth, we described a number of competence levels interacting with a number of domains or aspects of mindfulness-based teaching. A key question for us in developing the tool was: How many competence levels, and how many domains, can be observed both concurrently and over time?

We started out with 15 domains and gradually over time reduced the number to six. In earlier versions of the tool, agreement between assessors was low because it was difficult to discriminate between the domains. So we decided to reduce the number of domains, and acknowledged the multifaceted nature of each by defining key features that described and "unpacked" its various aspects. In practice, it is tremendously challenging (and ultimately impossible) to identify completely separate elements or facets of the teaching process. Nonetheless, while acknowledging the interconnection between the domains, we aimed to capture distinctive aspects of the teaching process with minimal overlap.

A particularly important principle was that the MBI:TAC needed to focus on quality, not quantity: we wanted the tool to assess the subtleties of competence and not simply be an elaborate adherence checklist. So, instead of simply assessing, for example, how often the teacher "expressed connection and acceptance" through how he or she related to participants, we felt it was crucial to attempt an assessment of how well the teacher conveyed these qualities. This required us to find a systematic way of describing competence levels within each domain. The MBI:TAC competence levels are based on the Dreyfus and Dreyfus (1986) model of skill acquisition and draw on the reinterpretation of this work by Sharpless and Barber (2009). Dreyfus and Dreyfus's landmark research on skill acquisition in a range of areas (airplane pilots, chess players, car drivers, and adult learners of second languages) demonstrated that the development of competence is a lifelong endeavor which continues to pass through subtle shifts. They suggested that people usually move through characteristic stages as they develop competence. Through systematic observation of the acquisition of mindfulness-based teaching skills in ourselves and in our trainees, we recognized these stages and were drawn to creating a tool that would describe a developmental approach to mindfulness-based teaching competence (R. Crane & Kuyken, 2012). We predicted that, given the right conditions (i.e., regular practice of teaching skills, regular engagement with daily personal mindfulness practice, attendance on retreats, appropriate training, and good quality supervision), teaching skills naturally develop over time. That said, it is of course also natural for there to be variation in the quality of teaching over time, and even within the same session.

Assessing Teachers' "Embodiment" of Mindfulness: A Particular Challenge

We have mentioned that our intention was that the MBI:TAC needed to focus on *quality* not quantity. We were acutely aware that, surrounding the explicit curriculum elements and themes, are interconnected implicit "curriculums" that are conveyed through the teaching itself, and are just as crucial to the overall learning process. Much of the learning is thus "caught" rather than systematically taught. Parker-Palmer (1983) aptly names this the "hidden curriculum" and argues that it needs to be intentionally designed and given as much attention as the explicit curriculum. The hidden curriculum is both subtle and powerful. The messages that are conveyed through *how* we teach embed themselves and influence attitudes, motivations, and behaviors in ways that words rarely accomplish.

So let us pause and bring to mind the nature of implicit aspects of MBCT teaching and learning. The MBCT learning process is founded on participants learning how to shift mode of mind from "driven-doing" to being (see Chapter 4). Through direct connection with the interplay of internal and external experience while residing in a "being mode, present moment, nonjudging" orientation, a fresh exploration of mind patterns becomes possible. Mindfulness-based teaching methodologies have developed precisely to create the conditions within which participants can cultivate being mode, and use this as an orientation from which to explore inner experience. A large part of this methodology is that the classroom atmosphere or climate itself offers an experience of mindfulness. It is the teacher who bears the prime responsibility for creating and sustaining this atmosphere, through his or her capacity to embody the qualities of mindfulness within his or her own being as he or she teaches. By "embodying" or "living" the principles of mindfulness throughout the teaching process, teachers offer participants tangible experiences of being in a mindful environment, so enabling the learning to "seep in." The learning themes are predominantly communicated implicitly through the process of the teaching. A teacher who has a strong capacity to embody mindfulness will communicate alignment between the implicit and explicit learning themes, so making it more possible for participants to connect with the learning.

Embodiment is thus an integral aspect of all mindfulness-based teaching and became one of the six domains in our assessment tool. Yet in developing the MBI:TAC, it was the embodiment domain that we found most challenging to capture through specific descriptors. We needed ways of describing what it "looks, sounds, and feels like" when teachers do the inner work of connecting mindfully to experience, and how this inner work is reflected in their verbal and nonverbal behavior. The key features of the embodiment domain that we arrived at, and excerpts from the MBI:TAC describing them, are presented in Table 16.1.

To recap, mindfulness is an internal process—a particular way of being in relationship with experience. In order to communicate this successfully to participants, teachers need to embody this process themselves. The term "embodiment" essentially describes how this interior work of mindfulness practice is implicitly reflected in the teacher's presence and behavior, influencing the atmosphere of the MBCT classroom. That is, embodiment reflects the extent to which teachers are mindfully connected with their experience and the interface between this, the group, individual participants, and the teaching process.

Implementing the MBI:TAC

The six competence levels and six domains of the MBI:TAC (R. Crane et al., 2012) are presented in Tables 16.2 and 16.3.

Table 16.4 shows a sample page illustrating how the domains and competence levels interact together. Each domain has a similar page, followed by guidance notes for assessors relating to each key feature. (See also the online full version at *http://mindfulnessteachersuk.org.uk/ pdf/MBI-TACJune2012.pdf*.)

TABLE 16.1. Domain 3 of the MBI:TAC: The Embodiment of Mindfulness

Key feature	Summary description
(i) Present-moment focus—expressed through behavior and verbal and nonverbal communication	The teacher offers a demonstration of present-moment focus so these are observable through their behavior and verbal and nonverbal communication. The expression of embodiment can be particularly sensed through the teacher's body—that is, their posture; physical groundedness and steadiness; physical sense of ease, calm, and alertness; steadiness; rhythm and pitch of voice tone; etc.
(ii) Present-moment responsiveness to internal and external experience	Evidenced by a relaxed calmness, together with alertness, aliveness, and vitality shown through language, bodily expression, and behavior. The teacher's sensitivity to personal direct experience directly informs their choices within the group. The teacher embodies a sense of "surrender" to the moment and to what is needed now. The teacher will use his or her attentional skills in both a wide- and narrow-angle way at different moments within the teaching.
(iii) Calm and vitality—simultaneously conveying steadiness, ease, nonreactivity, *and* alertness	There is evidence of the teacher bringing steadiness and calm along with an enlivened vitality and alert responsiveness to the moment.
(iv) Conveying the attitudinal foundations of mindfulness practice—nonjudging, patience, beginner's mind, trust, nonstriving, acceptance, and letting go—through the atmosphere created in the class	The attitudinal qualities that are inherent within the program are taught through embodied process throughout the teaching of mindfulness-based courses, as well as sometimes being conveyed verbally through interactive teaching. Participants are learning to learn in new ways through the modeling offered by the teacher of this way of being with experience.
(v) Person of the teacher—the learning is conveyed through the teacher's way of being	The teacher communicates through his or her way of being the essence of the learning process. How this happens is as individual as the person him- or herself. It includes a capacity to respond intuitively to the moment, to be with difficulty, and to appropriately bring live experience to the meeting with participants.

TABLE 16.2. MBI:TAC Competence Levels

Generic definition of overall competence level	Competence band	Numerical band
Key features are not demonstrated. The teacher makes consistent errors and displays poor and unacceptable teaching, leading to likely or actual negative therapeutic consequences. No real evidence that the teacher has grasped the fundamentals of the MBI teaching process.	Incompetent: *Absence of key features, or highly inappropriate performance*	1
At least one key feature present in most domains, but numerous substantive problems and overall lack of consistency require considerable further development.	Beginner: *Aspects of competence demonstrated but significant problems evident*	2
At least two key features at a competent level in most domains, but one or more major problems and/or significant inconsistencies that require further development. Teacher adequately takes care of participants' emotional and physical safety. Teacher would at a very basic level be considered "fit for practice" as coteacher/under supervision—the participants would not be harmed and are likely to have opportunities for learning.	Advanced Beginner: *Evidence of some competence, but numerous problems and lack of consistency*	3
Most key features are present in all domains, with possibly some good features, but a number of problems and/or some inconsistencies are present. Teacher demonstrates a workable level of competence and he or she is clearly "fit for practice."	Competent: *Competent, with some problems and/or inconsistencies*	4
All key features are present in all domains, with very few and very minor inconsistencies and evidence of good ability and skill. The teacher is able consistently to demonstrate these skills over the range of aspects to MBI teaching.	Proficient: *Sustained competence demonstrated with few or minor problems and/or inconsistencies*	5
Expected key features are present with evidence of considerable ability. The teaching is particularly inspirational and excellent. The teacher no longer uses rules, guidelines or maxims. He or she has deep tacit understanding of the issues and is able to work in an original and flexible manner. The skills are demonstrated even in the face of difficulties (e.g., challenges from the group).	Advanced: *Excellent teaching practice, or very good even in the face of participant difficulties*	6

TABLE 16.3. Summary Outline of the MBI:TAC Domains, the Overarching Domain Descriptors, and Their Key Features

Domain	Descriptor	Key features
1. Coverage, pacing, and organization of session curriculum	The teacher adequately addresses and covers the curriculum content of the session. This involves creating a skillful balance between the needs of the individual, the group, and the requirements of teaching the course. The teacher is well organized with relevant course materials and teaching aids readily available and the room appropriately prepared for the group. The session is well "time-managed" in relation to the curriculum. The session is well paced with a sense of spaciousness, steadiness, and lack of time pressure. Digressions are steered back into the session curriculum with tact and ease.	(i) Responsiveness and flexibility in adhering to session curriculum (ii) Adherence to the form of the program and coverage of themes and curriculum content (iii) Appropriateness of the themes and content (to stage of program and to the participants) (iv) Level of organization of teacher, room, and materials (v) The degree to which the session flows and is appropriately paced
2. Relational skills	The qualities that the teacher brings to participants and the teaching process mirror the attitudinal qualities that participants are learning to bring to themselves during the MBI program. Mindfulness is the awareness that emerges through paying attention to experience in a particular way: on purpose (the teacher is deliberate and focused when relating to participants in the sessions); in the present moment (the teacher has the intention to be whole-heartedly present with participants); and nonjudgmentally (the teacher brings a spirit of interest, deep respect, and acceptance to participants) (Kabat-Zinn 1990).	(i) Authenticity and potency—relating in a way that seems genuine, honest, and confident (ii) Acceptance—actively attending to and connecting with participants and their present-moment experience and conveying back an accurate and empathic understanding of this (iii) Compassion and warmth—conveying a deep awareness, sensitivity, appreciation, and openness to participants' experience (iv) Conveying genuine interest in each participant and his or her experience while respecting each participants' vulnerabilities, boundaries, and need for privacy (v) Mutuality—engaging with the participants in a mutual collaborative working relationship

(continued)

TABLE 16.3. *(continued)*

Domain	Descriptor	Key features
3. Embodiment of mindfulness	Mindfulness practice permeates the teacher and is expressed through two interconnected aspects to embodiment: "present-moment focus," and bringing the attitudinal foundations of mindfulness to moment-by-moment experience. Embodiment of mindfulness involves the teacher sustaining connection and responsiveness to moment-by-moment arising (within self, within individuals, and within the group), and bringing the core attitudinal foundations of mindfulness practice to all of this. These attitudes are nonjudging, patience, beginner's mind, trust, nonstriving, acceptance, and letting go (Kabat-Zinn, 1990).	(i) Expression of present-moment focus and attitudinal foundations of mindfulness practice through behavior and verbal and nonverbal communication (ii) Conveying present-moment responsiveness to internal and external experience (iii) Simultaneously conveying steadiness, calm, ease, nonreactivity, and alertness and vitality (iv) Conveying the attitudinal foundations of mindfulness practice through the teacher's way of being (v) Conveying "in the moment" (rather than focused on outcome) trust and confidence in the process of bringing mindful attention to experience
4. Guiding mindfulness practices	The teacher offers guidance that describes accurately what the participant is being invited to do in the practice, and includes all the elements required in that practice. The guidance enables participants to relate skillfully to mind wandering. The guidance suggests the attitudes to bring to self and experience throughout the practice. The practice balances spaciousness with precision. Skillful use of language is key to conveying all this.	(i) Language is clear, precise, accurate, and accessible while conveying spaciousness and nonstriving (ii) The teacher guides the practice in a way which makes the key learning for each practice available to participants (iii) The particular elements to consider when guiding each practice are appropriately present
5. Conveying course themes through interactive inquiry and didactic teaching	This domain assesses the process though which the course themes are conveyed to participants. These are at times explicitly drawn out and underlined by the teacher and at other times emerge implicitly within the process. The domain includes	(i) Supporting participants to notice and describe the different elements of direct experience and their interaction with each other; teaching themes are consistently linked to this direct experience

(continued)

TABLE 16.3. *(continued)*

Domain	Descriptor	Key features
	inquiry, group dialogue, use of stories and poems, facilitating group exercises, orienting participants to session/course themes, and didactic teaching.	(ii) Exploring the different layers within the inquiry process (direct experience, reflection on direct experience, and linking both to wider learning) with a predominant focus on process rather than content (iii) Teaching of themes conveys understanding of underpinning theoretical principles (iv) Teaching skills—teaching is concise, clear, participatory, playful, alive, responsive, and makes skillful use of teaching aids (v) Fluency—teacher conveys ease, familiarity with, and confident knowledge of the material
6. Holding of group learning environment	The whole teaching process takes place within the context of a group, which if facilitated effectively becomes a vehicle for communicating the universality of the processes under exploration. The teacher creates a "container" or learning environment within which the teaching can effectively take place. The teacher is able to "tune into," connect with, and respond appropriately to shifts and changes in group mood and characteristics.	(i) Creating and sustaining a rich learning container that is made safe through careful management of issues such as ground rules, boundaries, and confidentiality, but that is simultaneously a place in which participants can explore and take risks (ii) Clear management of group development processes over the 8 weeks—in particular management of beginnings, challenges from within the group, and endings (iii) The teacher consistently takes account of and responds to learning processes on a group level (iv) A leadership style that offers sustained "holding," demonstrating authority and potency without imposing the teacher's views on participants

TABLE 16.4. Sample Page of the MBI:TAC Illustrating How the Domains and Competence Levels Interact

Competence level	Example
	Domain 3: Embodiment of mindfulness
Incompetent	Embodiment not conveyed—for example, consistent lack of present-moment focus. Attitudinal qualities are not in evidence.
Beginner	At least one key feature adequate. Lack of consistent present-moment focus, or teacher not calm, at ease, and alert, or attitudinal qualities often not clearly in evidence—for example, teacher tends to default to seeing and working with things through their critical-thinking and problem-solving mind, or works in a goal-orientated way; lack of spirit of exploration.
Advanced Beginner	Several key features at competent level. Teacher does evidence embodiment of several principles of mindfulness practice within the teaching process but there is lack of consistency, or teacher demonstrates some skillful present-moment internal and external connectedness but this is not sustained throughout.
Competent	Most key features are present with an acceptable level of skill and some minor inconsistency; teacher generally demonstrates an ability to communicate the attitudinal qualities of mindfulness practice through his or her "way of being" in the areas of language, bodily expression, and behavior, and is mostly present-moment focused.
Proficient	All key features are present with a good level of skill—sustained levels of present-moment focus through the teaching and demonstration of the range of attitudinal qualities of mindfulness throughout with very minor inconsistencies.
Advanced	Teacher demonstrates exceptionally high levels of awareness of and responsiveness to the present moment throughout the teaching process, or works with high levels of internal and external connectedness. Attitudinal qualities of mindfulness present in a particularly inspiring way.

Assessors rate each of the six domains using a 6-point continuous adjectival tool of competence levels. A total score can be calculated by averaging the six domain scores, but often the tool is used to aid trainee development, in which case a profile of scores across each of the six domains is given. As we developed the domains, it was clear that each represented a distinct aspect of the teaching process; if any were not present, the teaching would have significant flaws and gaps.

Some are more substantial and multifaceted than others and we therefore defined them using more key descriptive features. Whether some are more important than others, however, is less certain, given that very little is known about which aspects of mindfulness-based teaching are critical in predicting participant outcome. This is an important issue for further research.

During the development phase, we discovered that assessors were using a range of approaches and methods to make their assessments. Some were directly "participating" in the whole teaching session (by watching a video as if they were present in the class), and then engaging in assessment, while others were employing a more "detached observer" stance. Our judgment was that this variability was likely to reduce interrater reliability. We therefore developed guidance on how to engage with the assessment process to ensure consistency of approach. Assessments are made by:

- Participating in the teaching (immersing oneself from a participant perspective).
- Making a global competence assessment anchored to global competence descriptors, in order to capture an overall view of the teaching.
- Making individual domain assessments anchored to key feature descriptors and competence level descriptors, so as to ensure that each domain and each key feature within each domain is represented in the assessment.
- Reviewing global and detailed scores alongside each other and checking out discrepancies by returning to the teaching recording.
- Recording the scores on a summary score sheet.

Thus, at different points in the assessment process, assessors are encouraged to move between deliberately giving primacy to "being mode of mind" (the intuitive experience of the teaching) and to "doing mode of mind" (the capacity to categorize, judge, and discriminate), and to deliberately shift their attention between a narrow and a wide focus. Assessors using the MBI:TAC need to be highly experienced in teaching mindfulness-based courses. This is because understanding the nature of competence in a particular intervention is best developed through training and experience in delivering the approach. Additionally, assessors require training in the use of the tool in order to ensure that they are using it in the standardized way. Finally, as many teaching sessions as possible should be viewed so as to ensure that what is assessed is a representative sample of the teacher's practice.

The literature on treatment integrity generally indicates that adherence and differentiation assessment do not require experience in the delivery of the approach because they involve a relatively simple checking of the presence and absence of intervention components. However since the MBI:TAC integrates assessment of adherence, differentiation and competence, assessors who are experienced teachers are required for the entire process. They need among other things sufficient experience to be able to judge whether departures from strict adherence to the program are appropriate or indeed necessary (e.g., when responding to the immediacy of the moment is prioritized over following the formal curriculum).

The MBI:TAC is now being used in the range of contexts in which the integrity of the mindfulness-based teaching is a central question. These include training programs and supervision during which the criteria are used as a developmental tool to offer clear feedback to trainees and to identify foci for development; university-validated training programs; and the selection and evaluation of teachers for research trials, where reliable and valid assessments of teaching integrity are crucial. As well as these examples of evaluation by another, the tool is also valuable as a self-reflective tool and aid to self-development, whatever teachers' level of expertise or stage of development.

There are challenges. Considerable effort and resources are required to assess teaching integrity adequately. However, our experience is that it is an invaluable learning process for those who submit their teaching for evaluation, and that it offers the clearest method developed so far of discriminating levels of teaching quality.

Research on the MBI:TAC

The MBI:TAC is the first tool that has been developed to assess MBSR and MBCT teaching integrity. Preliminary findings on its psychometric properties are encouraging (for a detailed report, see R. Crane et al., 2013). The reliability of the tool was evaluated during routine assessment practice in the three master's programs at Bangor, Exeter, and Oxford Universities where a proportion of student's teaching practice was independently assessed by two trainers. The overall intraclass correlation coefficient (ICC), which measures interrater reliability, indicated a good level of agreement ($r = .81$, $p < .01$). Even when assessors disagreed on one domain, the reliability of averaged ratings was excellent. Equally, the evaluations of validity that were possible at this early stage in the tool's development were encouraging.

Further research in a range of contexts is needed to clarify the MBI:TAC's reliability and validity. Research is also needed on the relationship between teaching integrity and participant outcome and on the effectiveness of methods used in training programs to develop core skills. The striking expansion of research on mindfulness in the last 15 years has predominantly focused on evaluating the outcome of mindfulness-based courses. There has been little research on the teaching/learning process through which these outcomes are achieved. Given that these processes are multidimensional, complex, and subtle, this is perhaps not surprising. However, developing greater understanding of how positive outcomes are brought about would be of great value in guiding future developments.

Concluding Remarks

Through using the MBI:TAC in practice, hearing from others who are using it, and from feedback at conferences and workshops, we have been encouraged to believe that it is making an important contribution to promoting best practice. This development has happened at a time of dramatic expansion in the interest in mindfulness and it is important that there are checks within the system to support the integrity of developments. We are convinced that the next phases of research and development will be full of discoveries, leading to refined versions of the MBI:TAC and to versions developed for particular contexts and mindfulness programs adapted for specific problem areas and participants' groups. We are also aware of the limitations of the MBI:TAC. *Descriptions* of phenomena are only that—descriptions—a finger pointing at the moon is not the moon. The MBI:TAC is a tool and, like all tools has useful applications and is good for certain jobs. We have noticed, for example, that the tool has a place within training, but that it can easily trigger in trainees ideas about what their teaching "should" look like—which runs counter to the predominant training theme of teaching from where you are in this moment.

It is important also to recognize that the MBI:TAC makes a significant contribution to ensuring the overall integrity of developments in mindfulness-based teaching, but is not in itself the whole story. In recent years, other contributions have added other important dimensions. For example, good practice guidelines for mindfulness-based teachers have been published in the United States and in the United Kingdom (Santorelli, Goddard, Kabat-Zinn, Kesper-Grossman, & Reibel, 2011; UK Network for Mindfulness-Based Teacher Trainers, 2011). These articulate the conditions within which teacher competency can grow. The specific aspects of the United Kingdom good practice guidelines that relate to MBCT ask that the teacher has:

- Knowledge of relevant underlying psychological processes, associated research, and evidence-based practice.
- If delivering in a clinical context, an appropriate professional clinical training related to the population that the group is being offered to.

The quality of mindfulness-based teaching is an important issue for the field. It is also a tremendously personal question that arises for every mindfulness-based teacher during the course of development. Because of the personal and intimate nature of the learning process, the doubts that inevitably arise about our own competence can feel painfully close to home. How we as teachers experience the teaching process from the inside is explored in the next chapter.

CHAPTER 17

The Experience of Being an MBCT Teacher

In Chapter 16, we highlighted the importance of delivering MBCT competently and as intended, and described the development of a measure that would enable reliable assessment of both of these priorities. All of us endorse the value of this stance, in the interests of offering our participants an opportunity to experience mindfulness that brings clarity and authenticity. When teaching within an evidence-based approach, however, what appears valuable (and indeed essential) to good practice may be experienced rather differently, as a pressure to perform well. Such pressure may take us far away from the spirit of nonstriving and acceptance that is cultivated in mindfulness-based approaches. The thought "I've got to get it right" may well come to the fore. These issues are particularly emphasized when the teaching is done within the discipline of a research trial, and especially when participants are as vulnerable to depression and despair as those we were working with.

In this chapter, we explore some of these issues from inside the "lived experience" of being observed. Teaching under close observation is challenging, but also offers a rare opportunity for sustained, clear-eyed reflection, which in turn can contribute to growing understanding of the qualities and characteristics of *all* mindfulness teaching. Specifically, the chapter considers how mindfulness teachers can support themselves so as to offer their best teaching. What are the circumstances and attitudes that help teachers to flourish? How can the human tendencies that might otherwise hinder this be worked with most skillfully, in order to develop and refine your teaching skills?

What Creates Skillful Teaching?: Doing and Being Modes of Mind

Mindfulness practice and learning to teach mindfulness share many processes that support understanding and choices about how best to respond at any particular moment. Reflective practice, based on both experiential and conceptual knowledge, offers both depth and breadth of view from which understanding can continue to develop. How does this happen?

In the United Kingdom, teachers of mindfulness-based interventions work within "Good Practice Guidelines" (*http://mindfulnessteachersuk. org.uk*) that define the range of knowledge, training, and experience required in order to become and remain a mindfulness teacher. The teacher's own meditation practice, supported by experienced teachers, given time to take root and become part of the teacher's life, offers a crucial foundation. All mindfulness teacher training programs require an extended period of established personal practice before considering offering this practice to others. This requirement reflects the shared and firm belief that skilled teaching arises only from personal practice. Direct experience of mindfulness meditation practice is essential to teachers' understanding of mindfulness, themselves, and the world. Time allows these understandings to go beyond a purely theoretical appreciation and become embodied and thus an integral part of *the being of the teacher.* The attitudinal qualities identified by Kabat-Zinn (2013, pp. 21–30) and the development and daily sustenance of mindful relationship to experience arise directly from regular personal practice; without such practice, no amount of reading, listening to lectures, or attending practical workshops will be sufficient. But having a personal practice is not itself sufficient. The skill of guiding others in a meditation practice, or holding a group of people as they then reflect on their mindfulness practice, demands different and additional skills and insights to those cultivated in regular personal practice. MBCT additionally requires an awareness of and subtle skills in teaching the carefully chosen cognitive exercises, which look deceptively simple, but are easily misunderstood.

As we described in Chapter 16, the MBI:TAC grew out of extensive discussions with training organizations in the United Kingdom and the United States, as well as discussions with colleagues in the rest of Europe. The MBI:TAC names a number of domains that characterize and so support skillful teaching. Some relate primarily to aspects of curriculum delivery: the "what" and "when" of teaching. Adherence to the MBCT curriculum means teachers delivering given exercises and practices in carefully chosen language and in a standard, carefully timed sequence that unfolds over the 8-week course. In part, the group is supported and nurtured by this clear and thoughtfully designed structure, which reflects a logical progression toward the ultimate intention of the course: acquiring the knowledge, skills, and compassionate, accepting stance seen as necessary to staying well.

"What" and "when" also covers the practicalities of teaching, for example, encouraging engagement and group development, and the organizational skills needed for both teacher and room to be prepared for welcoming participants to this particular learning opportunity. In some sense, the teacher here is making good and appropriate use of "doing"-mind (Chapter 4): aware that there are goals to be met in terms of what must be covered in the session, awareness of the clock, ensuring that the room configuration is as it should be, that hand-outs are prepared, and so forth.

Other domains described in the MBI:TAC reflect the "how" and the "why" of mindfulness teaching. These include relational skills; how teachers explore and invite experiential learning; and how their own practice is observably embodied in how they relate, pause, or choose questions in an inquiry process. These are the "being" aspects of mindfulness teaching, which would not be evident if teachers did not have an established mindfulness practice to draw on as they teach. Clearly, *doing* and *being* modes of teaching overlap and interweave. Understanding how this subtle, complex mix best supports skillful teaching and creates opportunities for learning continues to evolve and develop in the mindfulness community. The interrelationship between teaching skills and the emphasis given to each domain by teachers and trainers remains a fascinating area for further exploration.

For example, when a trainee is learning to teach mindfulness, initially "doing" aspects of teaching are usually given more prominence in the trainee teacher's mind and indeed in the training itself. New teachers want to know: "What am I supposed to do? When am I supposed to do it? How long should it take? And how do I actually *do* it?" They lean toward the "what" and the "when" of teaching and perhaps toward a sense of striving, needing to do things a certain way and to a certain standard (in which of course there is some truth). Trainee teachers learn how to deliver a particular exercise or practice, exploring different ways of expressing what needs to be said, staying within given structures and timings. They learn the order of the curriculum across a class and throughout the 8 weeks. They learn, for instance, that Session 2 generally starts with a body scan lasting 30–40 minutes, then an inquiry of around 10–15 minutes, then moves on to the home practice review and the first exercise designed to help participants understand the relationship between thoughts and feelings ("Walking Down the Street," Segal et al., 2013, p. 160.)

Understanding clearly the *why, how,* and *who* of teaching tends to take longer to develop, the connections arising gradually out of growing knowledge of and confidence in the more concrete aspects of teaching mindfulness. These are usually covered in the later stages of teacher training courses. Equally, it takes time and confidence to develop an authentic teaching voice, discovering who you are as a teacher. Many new teachers describe the initial challenge of bringing their personal mindfulness practice into the classroom, even when that practice is strong and well established. Bringing personal practice into the classroom does not mean "talking about your own practice." Rather, it means conveying the sense that the experiences and discoveries, the delights and the challenges, of meditation practice are shared by everyone in the room, including yourself as teacher. Bridging the gap between mindfulness for oneself and offering mindfulness to others is a significant (and sometimes unexpectedly difficult) process.

> Jo had had a committed daily personal practice for 5 years ahead of coming to a teacher training course. The early days of teaching practices were very challenging for her. She found it surprisingly difficult to guide practices using language that communicated her own felt experience of practice, tending to be very quiet in volume and using language that would mean little to newcomers to mindfulness. Jo's inquiry practices brought other challenges; her background as a therapist led her to ask questions that invited thoughts about the past rather than exploring the arising experience of the present.

What Jo was experiencing was the challenge of translating into words something that had previously been largely implicit and felt in her wordless inner experience. And this difficulty is particularly acutely felt if the teacher has long experience either as a therapist in another tradition or as an experienced practitioner of meditation and yoga. Both were true of Jo. Why, after years of confidently treating hundreds of patients and sitting hundreds of hours on retreat, should it be so difficult to teach a mindfulness curriculum? She was very frustrated. Surely her experience as therapist should have meant that she could see clearly and know how best to work with pain and distress in most of its forms. But as Segal et al. (2013) spell out with painful clarity in the book on MBCT for depression, expertise in one domain can make you blind to what is needed in another. For Jo, what made it doubly frustrating was that over the years, retreats had been for her a lifeline. She had sat retreats with many different and wonderful teachers, so how, she asked herself, could it be so difficult to lead a meditation practice? It is most confusing for us as new teachers. But perhaps it is not so surprising. Going to concerts to hear a great violinist may deepen our appreciation of music and perhaps increase our motivation to learn. Unfortunately, it does not give us the skills to play the instrument.

New teachers often initially describe feeling a mechanical and artificial switch between modes of mind. It can be hard to make the shift from practical doing-mind to a deeper felt sense of this moment, despite recognizing that this is the skillful thing to do. Practice in teaching, and yet more practice, is needed.

> Hannah described how as she first guided the body scan she would close her eyes in order to be in touch with sensations in her body to allow the language for her guidance to arise from her own experience but, also opening her eyes from time to time to check the time, ensure the volume of her voice projected sufficiently and to be in touch with the participants in the group as she guided them.
>
> At first, she felt that the "checking in" disrupted her guidance. Then she saw herself teaching on video and realized that the "switch" she felt to be disruptive "on the inside" was not discernible in the "felt quality" as it appeared on the tape. She realized that her *worrying thoughts about "checking in" were more interfering than the actuality of checking in.* Gradually, she was able to describe the fluent switch in

mode of mind as she opened and closed her eyes, sensing clearly the different ways that these supported skillful teaching.

As experience of teaching grows, these two ways of offering a class, both absolutely valid and necessary but in different ways, come to be accessed more easily and with more fluency. Choice grows in how best to respond to situations and experiences that arise in class, drawing from a broadening repertoire of skills and possibilities. As we shall see, ongoing teaching continues to require ongoing supervision or cosupervision, especially if you usually teach by yourself.

The Role of Supervision

Supervision plays an important role in supporting us in all types of mindfulness teaching, but especially in teaching that is being assessed because you are a teacher in training, or, as in our case, when our teaching was part of a research trial. During the research teaching, supervision was engaged with in different ways. As a teaching group, we "met" weekly for an hour to an hour and a half via teleconference to hear Mark's reflections on our teaching during the previous week's class, based on viewing video recordings of the classes. Geography did not allow us to meet so frequently in person, but we did meet in person as a teaching team, three times during each 8-week course. On each occasion, half a day of reflection and supervision ensured that we maintained protocol adherence and supported our development as teachers. Finally, we also occasionally met at each site separately to explore particular aspects of teaching and for reflection, trouble-shooting, and supportive guidance. This was supplemented by watching recordings of our own teaching and sometimes that of others in the teaching team. Finally, these processes were supplemented by regular, established supervision processes external to the research teaching teams.

Inskipp and Proctor (1995) described three roles of supervision:

- Restorative (supportive—to provide emotional and instrumental support where necessary).
- Formative (educational—to help develop and maintain skills).
- Normative (ethical—to maintain standards of adherence and competence).

In most supervision situations, one supervisor holds all of these roles, moving between the various functions at different points, creating whatever mixture is needed at any particular point. In some circumstances, however, these roles cannot all be held appropriately by a single supervisor. When the supervisee is being formally assessed, many training organizations require that the assessor is not also the supervisor. This acknowledges the potential conflict of restorative and normative roles. The research teaching team therefore felt that it was necessary to have a supervisor external to the research trial who was not responsible for the process of monitoring adherence and competence in our teaching. This parallels what happens in training courses in the United Kingdom where the roles of supervisor and assessor are kept apart.

Despite these cautions, the mode of mind taken into class by the teacher who feels under pressure to teach well because it is being assessed raises a number of issues, and it is to these that we now turn. Let us look at some particular examples of what can arise in the class.

What Makes a Skillful Teacher?

If you were teacher, how would you respond to the following scenario?

> In Session 2 of an 8-week MBCT course you are being video-recorded to assess your teaching competence. As usual, the video camera is pointing at you, and not at any of the participants, and because you yourself have probably just set it up, very much in your awareness.
>
> One participant, Bronwen, describes great difficulty in finding the time to do the body scan home practices. She says this in quite an angry way, complaining that it is impossible for anyone to find that amount of time and completely unreasonable of the teacher to expect this.

Take a few moments to imagine this scene. Allow your reactions to surface . . . what is it you'd like to say? Of whatever comes up, notice if any of it is associated with a sense of "being judged" as teacher, or a sense that you are being judgmental of the participant or wishing things were different at this moment. Notice any body sensation, especially any contraction or discomfort. Whatever mind and body reactions you notice, are they pleasant, unpleasant, or neither? Take a moment to acknowledge your reactions in an interested, friendly way.

There are always a number of options during any class. But the very same option may have a different "feel" if it comes out of a doing or being mode of mind. Doing mode can easily turn into driven–doing when you are anxious as teacher. In driven-doing mode of mind, you might react by becoming highly focused on the need for the group to be carrying out as much practice as possible, after all, "This should be done 6 days per week or people will fail to benefit." The focus is then on resolving this *difficulty*–perhaps offering suggestions about optimal times and places to get the practice done. The "just do it" message will come through strongly, and Bronwen may go away with some ideas about how to try harder or more effectively to make time for practice through the following week.

On the other hand, in being mode of mind, the teacher might first agree how difficult it is, and congratulate her for trying to do the home practice, then explore with Bronwen the processes she noticed when the idea of doing the home practice came to mind during the week. This would create a safe space for her to notice and become curious about whatever had unfolded. Taking time, the teacher could gently invite Bronwen to "unpack" what happened and at the same time to be closely attentive to her experience right now as they explore this experience. From this another kind of learning may arise:

> BRONWEN: It came into my mind that I had scheduled time to do the practice, but I had just too much else to do.
>
> TEACHER: Thanks, Bronwen. It sounds as if you were aware of the moment when you began to consider listening to the guided meditation and how, straight away, jobs that needed to be done arose in your mind? I wonder if you noticed anything in your body in those moments?
>
> BRONWEN: I felt tight and was thinking about all the marking that needed doing.
>
> TEACHER: So thoughts about work arose and your body felt tight. As you talk about this now, your head's lowered down and you're folding your arms. Is that where you felt the tightness?
>
> BRONWEN: Yes, it was. It felt like a load weighing me down—heavy

and tight across my chest. I had too much to do and the body scan was just another thing to be done. I felt angry then that I was being given something else to do when life is already too busy. Then I said to myself, "I can't do this. I'll go under if I try to do more. It's just not possible."

TEACHER: Ah yes. What you have described so well is just what we're asking ourselves to do in mindfulness—be aware of our experience and notice how it unfolds. You were practicing mindfulness as you were noticing these thoughts, sensations in the body, and emotions arising and unfolding. Were these thoughts and feelings ones that you recognized?

BRONWEN: Oh yes. I often feel like this. It's too much and I get fed up with people who add to the load.

TEACHER: And when you feel fed up what does that do to that feeling of heaviness and tightness?

BRONWEN: Oh, it grows bigger and then I can't do anything because I'm so wound up.

TEACHER: Thanks, Bronwen. (*to the whole group*) This is a great example of how our meditation practice is like a laboratory in which the old familiar patterns of mind show up. . . . Do you recognise any of this in yourself? We might even say that it's when the difficulties come up that the practice gets most interesting . . . so much to be seen and explored.

At this point it may well be important to remind participants of the importance of regular practice. But now it does not come out of judgmental reactivity as it might have earlier when you, as teacher, felt that your performance was on the line. Mere *instruction* to do home practice makes it sound as if it should be easy, and simply sets up guilt and resistance. Coming out of inquiry into the process, the next week's home practice comes as an *invitation* to do more investigation into familiar but potentially destructive processes. The home practice is now seen as *more* important because it is difficult. Rather than undermining the curriculum, the challenges have *become* the curriculum.

The various domains of the MBI:TAC identify the doing and being skills that are needed in order to teach with clarity and compassion. Teachers, their experience, and the unique set of circumstances present in the class at a particular moment will influence how far the teaching leans toward doing or being modes of connection and delivery. Many teachers describe times when they taught well seeming to arise as much by accident as by choice or design! Serendipitously, as it seems, a number of factors all came together and allowed skillful teaching to arise.

Responding to Moments of Discovery

A similar leaning toward doing or being might emerge in response to participants' positive experiences. Consider the following situation:

> In Session 5, after a sitting practice when the group were invited to bring a difficulty to mind, Eleanor described noticing sensations in her body more clearly than she had previously. She described the sensations that had arisen as quite intense as she'd brought her difficult situation to mind, but she had followed the guidance, heard the choices offered within it, and was able to stay with the heat, tightness, and "flashes" she had felt in her chest area. She had been surprised by the sense that arose that she could step back even from the powerful emotions arising from challenges in her life: that it was possible to feel this without being swamped by it.

Once again, take a few moments to imagine how, if you were teacher, you would respond. Allow your reactions to surface? Whatever comes up, notice if any of it is associated with a sense of "being relieved" that the participant is doing well and should be praised. Notice any body sensations. Whatever mind and body reactions you notice, are they pleasant, unpleasant, or neither? Take a moment to acknowledge your reactions.

Again, here is a point where a teacher might unwittingly slip from helpful, appropriate doing mode into goal-focused "driven-doing mode" (Chapter 4). A teacher leaning toward driven-doing mode might listen gratefully and with relief to Eleanor "getting it." He or she might recognize in what Eleanor said a series of useful teaching points, and (perhaps with a little impatience and concern about forgetting them if they are not named quickly) store these until the moment when they could be underlined for the whole group. Inside, the teacher might be delighted: "This'll be great on camera! What an opportunity!" And probably as these thoughts arise, the teacher has stopped listening attentively to precisely how Eleanor is describing her experience. As quickly as is polite, the teacher might thank her, and then proceed as follows: "Thank you so much, Eleanor, this is a great example, you are describing so well how if we stay with experiences, we might begin to see them differently."

Isn't it interesting how your attitude in these moments can reveal something about yourself: that what you think of as "openness and acceptance" as teacher can easily be *contingent* openness—you're open so long as the participants are making progress! You *like* how much you are being open—it feels so different from those times when you don't like what your participants are saying. In this positive mode, you may continue to name other learning for the group with a "smile to the camera." You are doing well!

The group may well hear the learning and take it on board, but perhaps more as an *idea* than through connecting to their own experience, felt in that moment in their bodies. But what on earth does it mean to "stay with" experience for those participants who have not had an experience remotely like this. For them, "seeing things differently" through "staying with" experiences remains meaningless. In the relief arising from your own unacknowledged doing mode (which loves "goals achieved" and "jobs done") you have not taken account of the pain of other participants who are at risk of feeling completely excluded from the celebration.

In being mode of mind this enquiry might feel quite different. The teacher might listen carefully to what Eleanor says and how she says it, creating space for her experience and allowing learning to emerge in the group. The confidence to do so relies on trust that learning will indeed emerge, patience to allow it to do so in its own way, and curiosity: How will this unique unfolding materialize in this class, right now?

In being mode, as Eleanor speaks, you as teacher are listening with care to what Eleanor is communicating. You may indeed be aware of the doing mode, in the back of your own mind, readying to congratulate and celebrate this moment of discovery. You see it clearly—you realize that the doing mode is here—that's fine—it is not a mistake. There is always something to celebrate—but you wait. There is a sense of "not yet." You decide to remain open and attentive to how the whole group are receiving her experience.

After some further enquiry with Eleanor about what she noticed in her body, from moment to moment, at this turning point in her practice, you see that there are several members of the group smiling and nodding in recognition. All in the group look interested in what Eleanor is saying. You as teacher feel able to broaden the discussion. This is how it might unfold:

> TEACHER: Do other people recognize this experience? (*People nod and smile.*) I wonder what your sense of this is—what's going on at these points? (*Asks the whole group.*) Would anyone like to say more?
>
> AMANDA: For me it is about letting go of being afraid of feeling bad. Not adding fear when I already hurt feels so different in my body.

As she says this she releases a big sigh and is visibly more at ease.

> ANNA: (*nodding and smiling at Amanda; holds her hand out gripping something imaginary in her palm and then turns the hand, palm upward, and slowly opens her fingers, as if releasing something*) Yes, it's good to let go of the tightness, isn't it?
>
> RICHARD: It's a bit different for me . . . just dropping in to feeling my body sitting here (*gesturing the body settling and connecting with his hands*) is such a relief compared to my usual way of thinking, thinking, thinking . . . "Why am I feeling like this? How can I make it go away? What's wrong with me? I can't handle this!", round and around. (*His hands are now up by his head making quick and circular movements communicating the busyness of this process for him.*)

The group are naming these experiences to each other, watching the way that these experiences are being communicated nonverbally just as much as the words being spoken. There is a sense of calm, surprise, and some excitement bubbling in the room.

TEACHER: I wonder . . . . what are you are noticing right now?

ELEANOR: It is exciting to feel that I can manage painful experiences when they crop up. . . . It's like I put my hand in the fire without getting burned! I didn't know I could do that. I feel really hopeful about the future!

TEACHER: Thanks. . . . and was anyone's experience different?

The teacher acknowledges that for those who have not spoken yet the meditation may have brought up very different experiences. Notice that the inquiry into difficulties and challenges is in principle the same as for more seemingly "positive" experiences: What did you notice—in the body, in thinking, in emotions, in impulses to act? The readiness to speak of difficulties, in the group or in pairs, is already a major act of courage for many participants. The "willingness to experience" is the feature that is being celebrated here. It is a reminder that each of us, whether in a mindfulness class or in our personal practice, are only responsible for the input, not for the outcome.

The teacher may end this inquiry by reading Rumi's "Guest House" and mention the possibility that arises out of mindfulness practice: learning to relate in new ways to the things in our lives that challenge us can seem hard, but it is helped by learning that there is something specific we can do: to be curious about what particular sensations are arising in the body, from moment to moment, when we notice we are in distress.

In teaching MBCT, as in other mindfulness-based interventions, all our different modes of mind are accessible to us as we prepare the room, gather people together, guide a meditation, listen deeply to the participants as they reflect on the practice done in class and at home, draw out any discoveries to be made from their experience, yet also answer their practical questions directly, and invite further observation as they take away the home practice assignments. The same curriculum element (e.g., inquiry in the examples above) can be delivered in many ways, depending on various factors such as the teacher's experience, temperament and state of mind, the unique characteristics of the group, and so on. The nature of the curriculum itself is another important factor.

The Role of the Curriculum

There has been some debate as to whether and how much the curriculum of any mindfulness-based intervention should be explicit or implicit. McCown et al. (2010) describe the "empty curriculum" of MBSR as necessary for the embodiment of mindfulness to be the primary way that mindfulness is communicated. In this context "empty" describes a way of delivering course materials that allows the curriculum to be introduced at the most appropriate moment for this particular group's learning. In this way, an exercise or the introduction of information can be offered at a point in the MBI program where this learning can best be received by the group rather than the teacher being guided primarily by the protocol. This may mean, for instance, choosing to wait until the following week to deliver an element of the curriculum if the teacher feels introduction of this element would create a disconnection from the learning that is emerging from experience in the class.

This is really important to bear in mind, alongside the realization that the essential structure of the foundational MBI curriculum (Kabat-Zinn's MBSR, 2013) has been tried and tested over more than 30 years. As McCown et al. (2010, p. 137) state, the many adaptations of MBSR that have emerged over the years all largely retain its structure and core practices (and this is true, for example, of MBCT). Teachers, new and experienced, trust in the scaffolding provided by this structure, and the way that it so skillfully unfolds over 8 weeks. The scaffolding instills a sense of ease and confidence, a sense of being safely held.

MBCT also offers a defined and structured curriculum that is designed to deliver the necessary components of the program, and has formed the basis for the current effectiveness evidence base. Core elements are clearly laid out and unfold intentionally, week by week, over the 8-week course. Learning builds on previous learning and materials are designed, based on experience and clear theoretical understanding, to offer opportunities to explore and develop learning for this specific client group throughout the course. The structure and manualized curriculum of MBCT have led some to suppose that emergent, experience-led learning is underprioritized in MBCT. Indeed, there is a danger that teachers are more likely too easily to switch gears to a didactic, lecturing style, for example, when they come to offer cognitive elements of the course or during the inquiry process, rather than realizing that this learning too can happen through experience and interaction. While it is crucial for the teacher to be clear about the intention of the practice or exercise in that moment of teaching, the need to explicitly name learning that might be available at this point, or to do this too soon, may unhelpfully tilt the emphasis too much toward conceptual learning and away from experiential discovery.

So is it a matter of simply either/or, structured curriculum or *empty* curriculum? Maybe the picture is actually more complex? It may be simplistic to say that an *empty* curriculum necessarily allows teaching to arise from the group, or that a *structured* framework will hinder this process. Some teachers may respond to the security of a defined curriculum, settling into being mode of mind as they teach, and would be challenged by a less structured curriculum. Perhaps this dynamic balance of structure and flexibility, of teaching from both doing and being mind, is a unique process for each teacher. Whether the curriculum is structured or more flexible, what arises in the class, between these particular people as they explore their particular experience, will be unique, emerging from moment to moment. The connection and responsiveness of the teacher cannot be planned or scheduled. Many trainee teachers name this as the predominant challenge of the inquiry process; without knowing what people will say about their experience it is impossible to have a defined plan to rely on. Here the teacher is held by their practice and willingness to not know and wait to see what emerges as experience is explored. But knowing the overall map of the mindfulness-based terrain is important. This includes both universal and specific aspects: How does universal suffering tend to express itself and how do any and all of us inadvertently maintain it. What is the specific intention of this practice used at this specific point in the program that helps us to explore this suffering wisely and in a way that is most transformative?

The Discipline of Teaching in a Research Trial

Teaching under close supervision, as in a research trial, where we are deliberately extending the range of MBCT, requires a particular focus on curriculum adherence. It is crucial that variables are limited where possible to allow change to be attributed to the elements being studied, which form the foundation of the MBCT evidence base. What is taught needs to be recognizably the MBCT curriculum and taught to an adequate standard. Otherwise the outcome, whether positive or negative, will be hard to interpret.

In trying to stay adherent because under close observation, it might be tempting to place greater emphasis on ensuring all the correct curriculum elements are present and timed perfectly than in many other contexts in which one teaches MBCT. Certainly, inclusion of required elements of the curriculum needs to be assured, and ideally the allocation of time to curriculum elements should be broadly similar from one research teacher to another. Yet what teachers actually do from moment to moment is and cannot be so constrained. The particular choice of language in practice guidance, the balance of fewer extensive inquiries versus more smaller inquiries to draw out key learning points—all these variables are under the control of the teacher as he or she discerns, moment by moment, what the class needs right now.

Teaching under the Spotlight

For both research and university-validated training, collecting the required information for assessment requires teaching to be observed, with a record kept for future reference by both the observer and the teacher. This process may involve video recordings, audio recordings or, at times, someone observing in person.

Usually, in order to support the teachers' development, these recordings are also available to the teachers themselves, allowing a partnership in the process of reflection on teaching. Processes of assessment of adherence and competence form the benchmark to inform, acknowledge skills and strengths, and support development where necessary.

There is an interesting pressure for most of us when teaching is assessed. When we began the research teaching for the trial in Bangor, we were surprised by the number of people who wished us luck. When people wish you luck you know something is up! This had never happened before for the many other classes we had taught under other circumstances. This teaching had a different sense of importance for us and also others around us. There was a sense of mindfulness itself (and the teaching team) being in the spotlight; the potential for learning and important additional understanding of this work to the mindfulness community.

Teaching that is leading toward a form of qualification or certification might have a comparable sense of importance. These very processes of observation and assessment almost inevitably instill a sense of vulnerability, maybe even threat. The fact that we want to be better teachers, and that we know that observation, assessment, and feedback are a valuable part of this process, does not make it any less threatening. Mindfulness teaching regularly happens in isolation; teachers may not regularly or frequently coteach or observe others teaching. They may talk with supervisors about the experience of teaching, and even perhaps belong to a supervision group, but this may not involve supervisor(s) directly experiencing and observing *their* teaching. You may have no idea how your teaching "compares to" other mindfulness teachers. Given the human need for approval and belonging, observation of teaching can stimulate a great feeling of vulnerability. This sense of vulnerability is perhaps heightened by the fact that mindfulness teaching requires the teacher's authentic presence as a mindfulness practitioner and as a person, moment by moment. These are important resources in teaching. So assessment of teaching is not merely an evaluation of knowledge and skill, but can seem as if it is assessing the teacher as a person.

Responding Skillfully to the Challenge of Being Assessed

Creating and maintaining an objective and sustained sense of the nature and quality of one's teaching is challenging, especially given the range of factors involved and the many alternative views possible as teaching is observed. Wanting to do well and to be seen as (at least) competent creates a sense of fragility, an uncertainty about the gap between where the teaching may be now, and how it needs to be. How do uncertainty and vulnerability impact on the teaching? How can you manage these processes so as to be able to teach well, even under these demanding circumstances? Consider the following situation that might be challenging for most mindfulness teachers:

> You are recording your class, or have a valued, experienced teacher watching you teach. One participant, Connie, has been reminded of her challenging parental relationship when she was a child. Thoughts of "failing to practice properly" have connected to other times when she felt a failure. Here, right now in the room, her memories and the connecting thoughts are fresh and present. She is telling the group details of a series of occasions when her father told her she was "useless." She is upset and appears to be lost in the familiar story as she replays these memories. She has told these same stories in at least two previous classes.
>
> The questions you ask to invite Connie to say what is happening right now in body and mind appear not to have been heard, and she is beginning another example. The rest of the group are getting impatient; this is a pattern for Connie they are now familiar with. They are looking to you to respond and continue with the class. You are very aware that this is taking a considerable amount of time, and worry that you won't have time to complete the required curriculum in the time allowed for the class.
>
> The potential for the whole group to learn from this situation may be apparent—but the most skillful way to respond right now is elusive. Maybe you are concerned that stopping her, even mindfully, will just add to her self-criticism and distress?

Take a moment to imagine this. What would be happening for you in this situation? Would this reaction be different if you were teaching alone, coteaching, or being assessed? And if so, what would make that difference? How much in the forefront of your attention would the camera/recording/observer be in this moment? Would you be prioritizing the observer, or Connie, or the group? The answer to these questions may make a significant difference to how you respond. With the observer in the forefront of attention, you may be focusing on doing well, getting this right, achieving. The meaning given to the observation, and perhaps the observer, may well influence the reactivity experienced in these circumstances. If, instead of focusing on the observation and the observer, it is possible to acknowledge their presence but allow them to be in the background rather than central in the field of awareness, then space becomes available to connect to mindfulness practice, the class, and the process unfolding. The conundrum of how best to respond can be held in mindful awareness, allowing a clearer view of this moment to emerge. Mindful awareness, in turn, opens up the possibility of conscious, wise choice in how best to respond. Here, creativity and flexibility will have the best chance to flourish. And this, after all, is precisely the transformative intention of MBCT.

Which of these teacher responses do you recognize as appropriate?

"Connie, it sounds as if there is so much going on at the moment, I wonder if I can ask you a question about it all? When these memories come back to you, what do you notice happens in your body?. . . . Is this happening right now?"

"[addressing the class] Connie's experience has raised a number of issues about how any of us cope when we get floods of memories coming back, and when it seems so overwhelming . . . can we divide into pairs and consider what each of us might do (or feel like doing) in this situation. First let's take a short breathing space."

"It's so difficult when these huge and painful memories come back so fast—it really seems the most important thing to do is to get rid of them or fix them in some way. . . . Let's take a breathing space to explore a different approach, impossible as it may seem."

"Thanks so much, Connie. There's so much here, and perhaps we can chat about it after the class [or 'come back to it later']. You mentioned how much of this is familiar to you, and I'd like to pick up on that . . . there are some practices that might help clarify things for us all—this next practice explores them more closely."

Even presenting these options can raise a sense of "there must be a right way to teach." This is not what we wish to imply. There are many different, equally skillful, ways of handing different classes, and each will have its unique consequences.

Teacher Doubts

It is a recognized phenomenon that learning a skill is often plagued by strong doubts about competence. It is appropriate that, no matter how experienced you are, if you stay open to learning, you will find yourself questioning your practice from time to time. But constant questioning can also hold you back. Palmer (1997) described a "sometimes crippling sense of fraudulence" that can arise. A sense of doubt and insecurity is a wholly normal stage in the development of any new skill. The problem for most mindfulness teachers is that many are learning these skills long after they have gained competence in other areas of their professional and personal lives. You might have been used to feeling unskilled when you first learned math or how to play a musical instrument, but to experience these feelings when you are "supposed" to be competent—this is a different matter. You can actually feel troubled, even resentful. And when teaching is under the spotlight of observation and assessment, these natural processes may inevitably come sharply into focus.

Are these feelings a barrier to your teaching, or might they be an ally? The internal processes that may occur as you are engaged in assessed teaching can offer valuable insight into the processes being worked with by MBCT course participants. There is a parallel process as you experience thoughts with high emotional content that draw you into their content easily and repeatedly. You can feel how you may be adding significantly to the pressure of being assessed through the thoughts you are having about being observed and the way you relate to these thoughts. Self-critical, judgmental commentary is familiar to mindfulness teachers: we know this well. Here is an opportunity to turn toward this experience in yourself and support yourself through practice.

Thought distortions show themselves:

"The assessor *is bound* to think this is not good enough." (Crystal ball gazing)
"This is probably the worst teaching they have *ever* seen and *everyone will know* this is so!" (Catastrophizing)
"I can't teach!" (Overgeneralization)
"This was a dreadful class." (The mind staying with the problematic aspects and missing the many aspects of that class that were skillful)

Through mindfulness practice, it is possible to become aware of an apparently continuous stream of comment and judgment about all aspects of experience. Sometimes, this monologue is valid and supportive, but often the judgments are habitual, skewed, unkind, and outdated. Think back to the scenario we asked you to envisage just now. What came to mind when you imagined having your teaching assessed by someone you respect? "Oh, good, I'm sure I'll learn a huge amount?" Or "Oh dear, what if they don't think I'm good enough?" The degree to which your internal critic and other thinking habits are present and active, and the sorts of things he or she may say, will be influenced of course by a number of factors. As cognitive theory suggests, thoughts about your teaching (like depressed thinking) will depend on mood, memory, your beliefs about yourself in a more general sense, and the meaning of the circumstances you find yourself in.

> Being open to the experience of feedback about your own mindfulness teaching is itself a mindfulness practice that will help to develop your skills more fully. The reflective process involves building new avenues of awareness and ways of seeing that support both personal and teaching practice.

In our work together in the Oxford–Bangor trial, we also found that being observed, watching our own teaching, and receiving feedback could give our internal critics considerable fuel. Who can honestly say that they welcome opportunities to record their teaching? It is frequently described as an aversive experience. As with all experiences that challenge where there is an element of threat, avoidance may arise for all of us. But we noticed that, over time, our willingness to watch recordings minute by minute, attending sufficiently closely and consistently to see the teaching in detail, evolved through the exposure we experienced during the period of teaching on the trial. The detail of notes taken reflects this clearly. The levels of curiosity, the questions being asked of the teaching, the awareness of where things were skillful and opportunities missed—all grew considerably as the levels of tolerance to the discomfort of watching ourselves teach increased. Awareness of the benefits of the process of reflection and feedback supported our willingness to be actively involved and to make the most of this opportunity.

What Can You Learn from Watching Your Teaching?

Feedback from others or through watching a video recording of one-self offer enormous possibilities for your teaching development. Being open to information about teaching helps to develop that teaching fully. The reflective processes involve building avenues of awareness and ways of seeing that feed into and support your personal practice as well. Over time, these reflective processes and the learning that emerges from them become more and more accessible during the teaching, rather than just afterward. Opportunities for teachers to work actively with their own difficult experiences inform teaching enormously, developing experiential wisdom from which trust in mindfulness practice strengthens. These experiences create a library of experiential knowledge that can be drawn on when working with challenge generally, and specifically in teaching. Here are several aspects that can be learned from watching your teaching (see also the sidebar on p. 279).

Grounding with Body Focus to Steady and Balance

Trust in the body as an anchor to return to in stormy moments offers grounded connection to this moment. Here you may witness again and again the power of *decentering to see your thought processes clearly.* There are many opportunities available to practice simply observing thoughts and the emotions, body sensations and behavior that are so closely connected to them. It becomes possible to see "teaching thoughts" clearly from a decentered, observational perspective rather than being caught up in their content.

Thoughts as Just Thoughts

We learn that we can choose not to follow their story, even if the emotional flavor is strong. We feel the power and energy of the pull of these thoughts arising just now—but we see this with kindness and confidence. They may be very familiar and simply *Territory of Being Assessed* thoughts just as in *Territory of Depression* thoughts. Of course you will feel like this, given these circumstances. Who wouldn't? This is just as it should be.

Broadening the View to Receive the Whole Picture

It may be true that some improvements or changes to your teaching might be helpful, or are even necessary, but it is equally true that some positive aspects of teaching will be evident too. The MBI:TAC has a summary sheet where both strengths and learning needs are recorded, underlining the importance of holding both in awareness as teaching is reviewed.

Choosing to Offer Yourself—and Your Patterns of Reactivity—Kindly Attention

As a mindfulness teacher you know that mindfulness is not about "fixing" problematic experiences, but as a human being the wish and urge not to feel discomfort is often strong. Here is an opportunity to practice acceptance and self-compassion, comforting and taking care of yourself as best you can during this challenging time, exactly because things are just like this at the moment.

JOSIE'S EXPERIENCE

Josie was training to be a mindfulness teacher. She described how she had been managing her stress around recording her teaching for a master's module at the university.

Josie: The moment that I saw that I was thinking "I shouldn't be feeling stressed about this" and I smiled at myself—this felt an important shift to me.

At that moment I saw clearly that it wasn't possible, given these circumstances, to feel anything other than stressed. I watched how my wishing it could be different led me to watching the gap between how things are now and how I wanted them to be. I talked to some of the other students and they were all feeling the same. Acceptance really allowed me to stop resisting and adding to my discomfort. On one occasion when I noticed I was having frightening thoughts about recording my class I did some yoga, which was just what I needed to be kind and to respond wisely to my tight body and the ruminative thoughts in my mind.

Seeing Different Aspects of Your Teaching

During the research teaching time on the Oxford–Bangor trial we were lucky that there was both time and encouragement to view and re-view DVD recordings of our teaching. There were some really interesting surprises in this work that, when we talked with colleagues, seemed to be shared experiences. One surprise was that our view of our teaching at the time of the class and the external, objective view captured by the camera seem to be regularly at odds.

We find a similar thing in our roles as teacher–trainers too. Especially early in their teaching development, many teachers describe a sense of busyness in their minds as they teach. There is a great deal to hold in awareness at the same time: timings of the class curriculum, themes for this part of the course, the experiences spoken about in the group, the nonverbal information being received and, of course, his or her own internal commentary, helpful or otherwise. This internal busyness is so vivid that it seems it *must* be apparent to participants and observing teachers. It is easy to assume that, because the mind is busy, it must seem busy in the room. Similarly, times arise for all teachers when they are at a loss for how to respond to a comment in the class or perhaps feel that they have not responded mindfully or skillfully. These moments may feel so emotionally charged that it is as if this, too, must be clear to all who can see.

To your surprise (and relief), you may often find that your internal sense of your teaching or the process in the class is not confirmed by either visual or auditory feedback. You may discover that, from the outside, there is considerably more spaciousness than feels present within you in those busy moments. The moment of "not knowing what to say" that at the time may have felt like it lasted for a long time might appear instead as a useful pause. Like us, you might observe that an emotion felt at moments of uncertainty or challenge is much less evident than you believed.

This is not to say that the internal sense of things is entirely unreliable, but rather that the tendency is to be alert to times when it seems the teaching has gone awry. The experiential knowledge that the sense of how things are going may in fact be biased can allow anxiety and doubt to dissolve a little, and even a sense of greater steadiness to arise. Here is a chance to see that thoughts are indeed not facts.

Watching recordings of teaching also allows an awareness of how perception and judgment of the teaching vary over time. In the class itself, often with the reviewer in mind, thoughts anticipating judgment of your teaching arise. Aspects of the teaching that are felt to have gone less well dominate the view of how the class has gone (as if we knew anyway). This can lead to a summary judgment such as "I didn't teach at all well in this class." Unsurprisingly, as thoughts do, this "hot" judgment will tend to initiate a series of thought processes elaborating the meaning and anticipated consequences of this "failure," with the connected emotion adding flavor. Any of us might get quite worked up in this situation and, in the middle of the night, feel like giving it all up.

Watching the class a day or two later can then be a surprising experience: things are likely not to be as catastrophic as you had believed. Interestingly, the relief at this point can mean that judgment becomes overly positive and aspects of teaching that can have been learned from the recording can be missed. So the outcome might be an equally biased view, but this time indiscriminately positive. There is a case to be made, at least once in a while, for several viewings of a single teaching session so that there is a chance for teaching to look different again. In time a much more balanced view, with a broader awareness of the range of material being seen, might emerge. A steadier, less threatened stance allows exploration, a chance to see things more clearly and from a more decentered perspective. The recording can be played and replayed to see details of the teaching. This can bring about a profound change in stance. What you are seeing becomes teaching, rather than *my* teaching. This in turn allows space to pause and see places where something happened in the class that had shifted understanding or opened up new possibilities. This fresh awareness is then really supportive in teaching the next session, offering new understandings that had been inaccessible in the full flow of the previous session. This process may be enhanced by using the MBI:TAC as a self-reflective tool, as we suggested in the previous chapter.

> There is a case to be made, at least once in a while, for several viewings of a single teaching session so that a more balanced view might emerge. A steadier, less threatened stance gives a chance to see things more clearly and from a more decentered perspective. This can bring about a profound change in perspective. **What you are seeing becomes teaching, rather than *my* teaching.**

The opportunity for another teacher—an objective other—to watch teaching (and perhaps assess its integrity and quality) can sidestep this lengthy process. Without the same emotional connection to the material being watched, a clear view of teaching may be accessed more quickly. Someone else will almost certainly offer a slightly different perspective or viewpoint, giving breadth and depth to the teacher's own understanding as they see more or different aspects of teaching. The challenge of having one's teaching observed and/or assessed is balanced by the clear benefits gained.

Concluding Remarks

So assessed teaching is a challenging practice. How can you best support yourself through this process? How can you manage your sense of threat and anxious thoughts about observation and assessment, the urges to avoid that are triggered, the resistance, or getting lost in elaboration that may arise? How can you maintain creativity and stay in connection with the precious resources offered by the being mode of mind?

Teaching practice, like personal practice, offers ways to hold experiences with kindness and sensitivity, reminders to create space enough to respond as wisely as possible. Repeated practice, and later reflection on it, allows choices to become available, enabling unsupportive thoughts and video cameras not to be in the forefront of attention. It becomes possible to focus on what is actually here in the present moment, rather than on what might happen. Gradually, you will find that the process of reflection on your teaching allows and accepts the presence of challenging experiences in awareness, welcoming them as opportunities for learning and practice. If we appraise circumstances as simply "fine," although this may be comfortable, it rarely fosters motivation to explore and further develop understanding and skills. Learning to teach mindfulness is an extraordinary privilege, and it involves working at an edge. This can be challenging, but it is often these "edges" that allow greater awareness to open, new horizons to be seen.

PART IV

MBCT— THE RESULTS

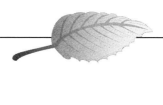

CHAPTER 18

Mindfulness on Trial

Does MBCT Help People at Risk of Suicide?

The focus of this book has been on how we may best help reduce suffering for those who suffer repeated episodes of depression, and who become acutely suicidal during these episodes. We have seen that this group of people are at highest risk of eventual suicide or serious suicidal behavior. There are a number of factors that put them at risk: their depression is more likely to run in families (Kendler, Gardner, & Prescott, 1999); they are more likely to have suffered adversity and abuse as children (Brodsky et al., 2001), and to have acquired a number of different mental health diagnoses over their lifetime, reflecting the uncertainty of physicians about how best to help (Oquendo et al., 2005). Yet little is known about how to prevent suicidal crises in this group.

The fact that depression is often a chronic relapsing condition, with relapse rates of over 50% in those who have been depressed before, is particularly problematic for those who become suicidal when depressed. Our early research at Oxford showed that if suicidal ideation occurs during one episode of depression, it is a more persistent feature in later episodes than any other noncore symptom of depression (Williams et al., 2006). The habitual recurrence of suicidal thoughts makes them more accessible when mood plummets, increasing the chances of further suicidal crises (Joiner et al., 2005). This makes the question of how best to prevent the recurrence of depression particularly urgent for patients who habitually become suicidal when depression returns.

In Part I we explained how our early research helped us to understand suicidality better: we pointed to a phenomenon called "solution blindness" and suggested that some people are extremely susceptible to such a mind state. For some, when mood begins to lower, old patterns of thinking and feeling reemerge that bring a sense of defeat and entrapment, and severe mental pain that feels intolerable and unremitting, ending with suicide or self-harm as its visible expression: the cry of pain. What we see is a sudden collapse in confidence, a withdrawal, a breakdown in ability to think straight and solve common problems, a massive sense of exhaustion, and a deep need to give up. Because depression already makes a person vulnerable to several aspect of this pattern (especially fatigue, low energy, difficulty concentrating, lack of enjoyment of things that used to be pleasurable and nourishing) then it is most commonly during episodes of depression that such entrapment, self-harm, and suicide occurs.

For most people, suicidal thoughts and images are immensely distressing and they would do anything to avoid them. For a minority, however, they are comforting; they contain the escape from pain that is most desired. Catherine Crane made a special study of such "comfort" aspects of suicidal thoughts. She found that people who reported their images and thoughts as most comforting had in the past experienced more serious suicidal urges and behavior. However, even when taking into account these historical factors, those who found the idea of suicide comforting at the beginning of the research experienced the *worst* recurrence of suicidal mood over the next 12–18 months. Comfort is no protector from the extreme mental pain of entrapment (C. Crane et al., 2014).

Previous Research on Preventing Relapse in Depression

While antidepressant medications remain the most widely used treatment for depression, the high risk of relapse or recurrence after stopping medication has been the motivating factor in our search for a new approach to preventing depression. Before we started our Oxford research program to understand and prevent suicidal depression, only one trial had shown that MBCT, offered when a patient is in remission, was more effective than usual care as a preventative approach (Teasdale et al., 2000) and another was *in press* (Ma & Teasdale, 2004).

But there was a puzzle in the results of these two studies that was not clearly resolved. Both divided up the group of participants before they were randomly allocated to receive either MBCT or usual care (called "treatment as usual" [TAU]) by the number of previous episodes of depression they had experienced (two vs. three or more). This is called "stratification," and the reason for doing it is to ensure that each arm of a trial has approximately equal proportions of people who are (or are not) vulnerable and therefore may be responsive or nonresponsive to treatment. These studies predicted (and indeed confirmed) that those with more previous episodes were more vulnerable to relapse, so stratifying before randomization on number of prior episodes made good sense. Most studies of psychological treatment find that people with the longest history of psychological problems, and the more episodes of breakdown, are the *least* responsive to a new treatment. Things tend not to work for them; they haven't worked in the past—they don't work in the future. With MBCT, the results were exactly the other way around.

Both studies found that while MBCT reduced risk of recurrence in patients with three or more prior episodes, for patients with two prior episodes (the minimum required to be recruited to the trial—around one fourth of the sample) there seemed to be an *increase* in depression recurrence following MBCT, compared to TAU. While this increase was not statistically reliable in either study, when they are combined by meta-analysis, it becomes marginally significant ($p = 0.07$; Piet & Hougaard, 2011). As a result, subsequent studies on the prophylactic effect of MBCT have focused only on patients with three prior episodes. This seems straightforward and sensible, but in fact things are not so clear. Ma and Teasdale (2004) concluded that the number of episodes in itself may *not* in fact be the most important distinction between these groups. But if the number of previous episodes is not the critical determinant of vulnerability, what is? Unless we clarify this question, we will not discover for whom MBCT is most effective.

As we have said, Teasdale et al. (2000) and Ma and Teasdale (2004) had stratified their sample by number of prior episodes on the basis that this variable was a known predictor of relapse and recurrence. However, both studies found a number of *other* important differences between the groups. First, those patients who experienced three or more episodes had an *earlier age of first onset* of major depression, so that their total length of history of depression was considerably longer than those with only two prior episodes (20 years vs. 5 years). Second, Ma and Teasdale (2004) showed that if depression recurred for those patients with only two prior episodes, it was more likely to follow a major life event. By contrast, a recurrence in those patients who had three or more prior episodes was more likely to have no detectable precipitating life event—to be *autonomous*. These data were consistent with the original intention for MBCT, developed as it was from a model of cognitive vulnerability to depressive relapse (Segal et al., 1996; Teasdale, 1988; Teasdale et al., 1995) that assumed that ongoing vulnerability to depression was dependent on the patterns of negative thinking that become reactivated by relatively small downturns in mood (Ingram, Miranda, & Segal, 1998; Segal, Gemar, & Williams, 1999).

Yet here too it is not just the number of episodes that is important. Kendler, Thornton, and Gardner (2001) suggest that some people are vulnerable even before the first episode. That is, there are some who need fewer major life events to trigger even the first major depressive episode, due either to genetic vulnerability or to a history of adversity and trauma in childhood or adolescence. These results suggested a wholly new possibility: that MBCT works for those whose high reactivity to low mood arises not through repeated episodes of depression, but for those whose reactivity (and thus vulnerability) has been present since childhood and adolescence due to genetic/temperamental factors, or to a history of adversity or trauma.

Consistent with this finding, Ma and Teasdale (2004) showed that people with three or more episodes had significantly more adversity in childhood and adolescence. Using the Measure of Parenting Style (Parker et al., 1997) that had been validated against psychiatrist's ratings of patient's abuse experience recorded during clinical interviews, Ma and Teasdale found that patients with three or more prior episodes reported more abuse and more indifference from their parents prior to age 16 years. Those with only two episodes prior to the trial were no different in reports of parenting style from a "never depressed" control group. Ma and Teasdale (2004) conclude that these two groups (two vs. three or more prior episodes) were not simply members of the same population of depressed patients who happened to be referred for help at different points in their lifetime of recurrent depression, but might represent entirely different *types* of depression due to biological differences, or differences in childhood experience.

The anomalous results were to continue as we embarked on our program of research. Although Godfrin and van Heeringen (2010), working in Belgium, found a reduction from 68 to 30% recurrence over 12 months following MBCT (compared with TAU in those with three or more episodes), Bondolfi et al. (2010) did not replicate this result. Their Swiss study found that the "control group" receiving treatment as usual had a considerably lower risk of relapse in the follow-up period (34%) than that reported in earlier trials (66%, in Teasdale et al., 2000; 78% in Ma & Teasdale, 2004). With such a low "natural" recurrence rate, it was going to be very difficult for MBCT to make a difference. This is exactly what they found: although MBCT delayed the onset of a new episode of depression by 19 weeks, by the end of the 1-year follow-up, there was no overall difference in proportion of people who relapsed following MBCT versus the TAU control group. Bondolfi et al. explained the better than usual outcome in their control group as perhaps due to advances in standard treatment protocols for major depression, with Switzerland having high accessibility and availability of mental health care. An alternative explanation was that the cohort they studied were simply not as vulnerable as those of earlier studies, despite having experienced three prior episodes. A pattern was beginning to emerge: it seemed as though MBCT might work for those who, for some reason, had a naturally high risk.

Another important study by our colleagues in Toronto was soon to confirm this pattern. Segal et al. (2010) reported no overall improvement in recurrence rate for either continued antidepressant medication or MBCT for the *less* vulnerable patients in their study (i.e., those with *stable* remission in response to medication), despite this group having experienced three or more prior episodes. "Remission" refers to a period of time when symptoms of an illness have receded, but have not receded for long enough for a person to be sure of "recovery." In Segal et al.'s study, *unstable* remission meant that one week the symptoms would seem to have disappeared, only for them to reappear the next. All patients in their study had three or more previous epi-sodes, yet remission was unstable in some patients and not in others. Those whose pattern of remission was unstable had a higher risk or recurrence.

These results were fascinating. The relapse rate for patients with *stable* remission following initial successful treatment with antidepres-sants, but then no further active treatment (the placebo condition), was approximately 50%, and neither MBCT nor continued antidepres-sants made any further difference. For those with *unstable* remission, however, the relapse rate for those receiving no active treatment was close to the findings of original studies (71%), confirming that these were the more vulnerable patients. For these *more* vulnerable patients, both MBCT and antidepressants had a significant preventative effect, reducing the rate of depression relapse to 27% and 28% for the medi-cation and MBCT groups, respectively.

This pattern of results from five different studies would have severely limited the applicability of MBCT were it not for the sugges-tion that *the type of person for whom MBCT is most effective is the one that is normally most difficult to help*: those with *earlier onsets* and *more prior episodes* of depression, whose *remission is unstable,* and who have a *his-tory of adversity and trauma.*

Within our own program of work, we now had the chance to examine not only whether MBCT would reduce risk of depression in people at risk of suicide, but also to see whether each of these four aspects of vulnerability also influenced the effectiveness of MBCT in such patients. In the light of the evidence that depression is the final common pathway for around 80% of serious suicidal behavior, we wanted to focus our attention on whether MBCT would reduce the risk of another episode of major depression. If we could reduce risk of depression, we would be able to offer hope for these people who were at high risk. But, given our interest in the *reactivation* of suicidal ideas when people get depressed, we also wanted to see if, after MBCT, participants—even if they experienced low mood in the future—might do so without the mood re-creating old patterns of suicide and self-harm. For many clinicians and researchers, this is the "holy grail" of suicide research. Why? Because we cannot hope to ensure that our most vulnerable patients never get depressed again. A major break-through would be made if we could find a way so that people, even if they became sad, low, or depressed, would be able to do so without feeling suicidal. But there was another question that is often raised when the results of MBCT are discussed: How do we know that it is the mindfulness that is the active ingredient?

Is It Really Mindfulness Meditation That Is Critical?: The Need for an Active Treatment Control

Despite there being many studies across the world that show that MBCT can prevent depression in vulnerable patients, there is one aspect of MBCT that no study had yet addressed: the issue of nonspecific factors. Nonspecific factors are those aspects of any intervention that are present whatever treatment is offered: support from a therapist or teacher, support from a group of people with similar experiences, psychological education about mental health issues in general and depression in particular. No study had used a group intervention comparison condition, matched to MBCT for exposure to a teacher and group support, and for the psychological education about depression and how to meet it that the classes involve. No study therefore had been able definitively to attribute the beneficial effects of MBCT to its specific components rather than to these more nonspecific factors.

The Choice of Comparison Condition

There are several options when selecting a "control" treatment. We could compare the MBCT "package" with an alternative group-based package, for example group-based CBT that would entail comparable group attendance and homework assignments. There are two reasons why we rejected this option. First, treatments like CBT were designed to treat acute depression rather than prevent relapse, and appear to be less effective in preventing relapse when used as a preventative approach (Bockting et al., 2005). Second, whatever the outcome of such a comparison, we would be unable to answer our key scientific question: Which component of MBCT is critical to success? We decided to use a "dismantling" paradigm in which the comparison treatment is identical to MBCT, but has a critical component—training in meditation—removed. We called our comparison treatment cognitive psychoeducation (CPE). In CPE, participants would have the same number and length of sessions as those in MBCT, so receive the same group and teacher support, but instead of meditation training, they would receive information about depression, and do practical exercises within and between sessions inviting them to apply what they were learning. Group discussions would cover the psychoeducational components of MBCT: learning about depression, links between thoughts and feelings, and how to self-monitor these for signs of impending relapse.

Calling in Help from Bangor

As is now clear from reading this book, the Oxford University research group could not do this alone. In order to test whether MBCT would be able to reduce depression in patients who were now in remission (feeling better), but all of whom had experienced three or more episodes, we would need around 300 patients in a randomized controlled trial. Mark Williams contacted Professor Ian Russell, his successor as director of the Institute of Medical and Social Care Research at Bangor University in Wales, and Rebecca Crane, the director of the Centre for Mindfulness Research and Practice at Bangor, to explore if they might collaborate in running a two-center trial that would form an extension to Mark's next Wellcome Trust-funded Oxford program. Bringing the Oxford and Bangor teams together had many advantages beyond the obvious attraction for Mark of working with many of the very colleagues and friends who had shared in the early implementation of MBCT in the United Kingdom. Ian Russell was an expert on randomized controlled trials. He and his wife Daphne Russell are trial statisticians, experts in a very specialist field that has moved far beyond the statistics that most psychologists learn as part of their training. The Centre for Mindfulness Research and Practice in Bangor, led by Rebecca Crane, had become a premier center for MBCT training in Europe and beyond. Here was a concentration of skilled mindfulness trainers dedicated to cultivating, extending, and deepening the practice and teaching of mindfulness, and committed also to helping the evidence base for mindfulness to grow even further. In Oxford, Melanie Fennell and Thorsten Barnhofer would teach classes, and Catherine Crane and Danielle Duggan would oversee and manage the trial on a day-by-day basis. For the trial itself, we expanded the Oxford research team to include Ann Hackmann, Kate Brennan, Dhruvi Shah, Kate Muse, Adele Krusche, and Isabelle Rudolf von Ruhr. In Bangor, Rebecca Crane and Sarah Silverton joined the team as teachers, with Mariel Jones and Elaine Weatherley-Jones as recruiters and Catrin Eames and Sholto Radford as research assessors. The North Wales Organisation for Randomised Trials in Health (NWORTH) would be responsible for randomization of participants using computer algorithms, and later, Chris Whitaker and Yongzhung Sun would begin the complex task of analyzing the data without reference to the main research team, who were to remain completely blind to the results until the primary analyses had been completed, after which Daphne and Ian Russell would be there to help conduct the final statistical analysis.

Whom Did We Invite to Take Part in the Trial?

We recruited participants through referrals from primary care and mental health clinics in Oxford, England, and Bangor, North Wales, and through advertisements in the community. To assess their history of depression, we used a "gold-standard" diagnostic interview: the SCID (First et al., 2002). To be eligible for the trial, participants had to:

- Be between 18 and 70 years of age.
- Have a history of at least three prior episodes of major depression, of which two must have occurred within the last 5 years, and one within the last 2 years.
- Have been well ("in remission") for the previous 8 weeks.
- Be willing to give their informed consent and gain the agreement of their primary care physicians for their participation.

Prospective participants were not included if they had a history of the following diagnoses: schizophrenia, schizo-affective disorder, bipolar disorder, organic mental disorder, or pervasive developmental delay; if they had a primary diagnosis of obsessive–compulsive disorder or eating disorder, currently abused alcohol or other substances or regularly self-injured (e.g. cutting or burning) that was not associated with suicidal thinking. Due to the known effects of CBT in reducing risk of relapse, we also excluded those who had received treatment with CBT and had suffered no relapse to depression since treatment. They were allowed to join the trial if they had had CBT and then relapsed. Other reasons for not being able to participate were (1) if a person was currently receiving psychotherapy or counseling more than once a month; (2) if a person was practicing meditation regularly (i.e., more than once per month); or (3) if they could not complete research assessments through difficulty with English, visual impairment, or cognitive difficulties. The number of participants recruited was 274 (see the sidebar below).

One of the first things we looked for in our data, even before the trial started, was the age of first onset of major depression in our sample. Zisook and colleagues (2007) had found that, in adults coming to clinics for treatment of depression in a large U.S. study, careful interviewing revealed that the most common age for major depression to start was between 13 and 15 years of age. Their interviews took place when people were feeling depressed, so there is a chance that the results might have been biased by mood. Many people, when they feel

TRIAL PARTICIPANTS

- 274 participants recruited.
- Mean age of 43 years, *SD* = 12 years (range 18 to 68).
- 198 (72%) female.
- 13 (5%) describing themselves as non-Caucasian.
- Numbers analyzed = 255/274 (93%)
  - MBCT; N = 99
  - CPE; N = 103
  - TAU; N = 53
- MBCT: 89 (90%) of participants completed four or more sessions
- CPE: 97 (94%) completed four or more sessions.
- Median number of treatment sessions attended was seven out of eight in both treatment arms.

down, are inclined to say "I've always been like this," so it is possible that people's sad mood exaggerated early onset in their study. We had recruited people who had been depressed in the past but were now well. Would we find the same results when mood biasing of memory was less likely to occur? Figure 18.1 shows our results, virtually identical to the Zisook study.

A small proportion could not recall a time when they were not depressed, but the main results showed that half of our recurrently depressed adults had become depressed for the first time before the age of 18. Once again, *the most common age for the first episode of depression occurred between 13 and 15 years of age.* The earlier that depression first occurred, the more likely it was that the person had suffered childhood trauma and abuse and, unsurprisingly, the more likely that he or she later experienced suicidal urges and behavior.

Against this background, we recruited participants into the trial and randomly allocated them to receive either MBCT, CPE, or TAU. Nineteen (7%) subsequently left the trial, so the data analysis focused on 255 (see the sidebar on p. 294).

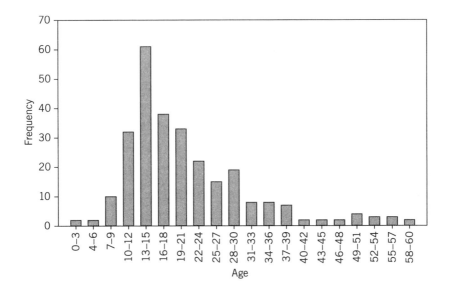

FIGURE 18.1. Age of onset of first episode of major depression. From Williams et al. (2012). Reprinted with permission from the authors.

Treatment Credibility

There is a well-known phenomenon in clinical trials in which participants tend to do better when given a treatment that they think is plausible, that suits their own ideas about what is causing their distress and
the best way to deal with it. This is really important if one is comparing
two different treatments. If one is perceived as more plausible than the
other, then any differences between the two might not be due to the
treatment actually being more effective in itself, but simply to the fact
that it *seems* more credible, and therefore motivates people more to
engage and stay the course.

To take account of this, all participants that were allocated to
MBCT or CPE rated the credibility of their allocated treatment at the
start of Session 2 on three scales from 0 to 10. The pattern of scores
showed that CPE was slightly more credible than MBCT, but not significantly so (see the sidebar below). The lack of a difference between
the MBCT and the CPE groups suggested that, should one treatment
prove more effective than the other, it would be unlikely that this was
because of a difference in credibility.

What Did We Find?

Our primary outcome was time until relapse to major depression over
the following 12 months. We defined "relapse" as meeting relevant
diagnostic criteria for major depression for at least 2 weeks. Participants were interviewed before and after treatment, then on four further occasions every 3 months during follow-up. To check that we were
assessing relapse to depression accurately, two independent psychia-
trists listened to audiorecordings of a sample of 91 follow-up clinical

---

TREATMENT CREDIBILITY QUESTIONS
(0–10 SCALE)

1. Expectation of treatment success (MBCT = 7.3; CPE = 7.9)
2. Plausibility (MBCT = 6.2; CPE = 6.6)
3. Would you recommend it to a friend? (MBCT = 6.7; CPE = 7.1)

interviews to reassess them. They rated an equal number of "relapse" and "no relapse" interviews, and we found a very high (87%) level of agreement on whether relapse had occurred.

Before the research team had sight of the data, the statisticians conducted the analyses that had been planned. They found that, regardless of treatment received, there were some participants who, as predicted, were more likely to relapse than others: those who started the study with unstable remission (i.e., still experiencing residual symptoms of depression) and those who had a history of childhood trauma. Even at this stage, however, the statisticians could see the same pattern that other studies had found before, that the two active treatments did not seem to have produced an overall reduction in relapse. The raw relapse rates for the 255 participants with follow-up data were 46% in one group, 50% in another group, and 53% in the third group. These differences were not statistically significant. But the statisticians had also conducted a planned analysis to see whether the indicators of vulnerability from previous trials (number of prior episodes, age of onset of first depression, unstable remission, and childhood trauma) influenced whether Treatment A or Treatment B (without knowing which was which) was more effective for the more vulnerable, and were able to identify which factor was most important.

The results were very clear. They reported to the team that they'd found that three of the indicators of vulnerability (age of onset, number of episodes, and instability of remission as indexed by residual symptoms at the start of the trial), had *no* influence at all in determining the effect of treatment. Only one factor stood out when all were put into the analysis: childhood trauma. One of the active treatments was having a much bigger effect than the other, depending on the level of trauma, but neither the statisticians nor the research team knew which treatment this might be: CPE or MBCT. This was because the analysis had been done "blind" by the statisticians, as mandated for the proper conduct of trials, and, of course, the researchers had taken no part in the analysis at all.

We held a trial steering committee meeting in which the overall pattern of results was reviewed. We could see the interaction, but did not know what results were behind it. We took the unusual step of deciding that we should not yet reveal to ourselves which group was showing which pattern, but instead asked the statisticians to continue to analyze the data blind, but this time to split the groups into high and low child trauma, so we could see the pattern of results for each treatment for each level of child trauma. We agreed to meet up again 3 weeks later to see what was going on.

So our colleagues went away to conduct further exploratory analyses, splitting the sample at the median childhood trauma score (median = 39.00) into high ($n = 126$) or low ($n = 129$) scorers, and examining the effect of treatment group (A or B) on the risk of relapse for each subsample.

When we met again, we saw the data in Figure 18.2. We could see which group the TAU group was (because it had half the number of participants)—and we could see that for the most vulnerable participants it was not doing very well. The graph in Figure 18.2 is a "survival curve" in which each deflection downward represents another recurrence of depression. Whichever group was on the bottom line was doing worst, with the highest probability of relapsing back into depression. Those on the top line were relapsing least. There were some clear differences emerging.

We decided it was time to discover which treatment group was which. Chris Whitaker had taken responsibility for the analysis up to this point, and he had with him a sealed envelope that would reveal to us all which was MBCT and which was CPE. Once the envelope was opened and the code was broken, we all saw that, for the most vulnerable people with a history of childhood trauma, it was MBCT that was the most effective in reducing relapse. For these participants, the pattern for MBCT versus TAU almost exactly replicated the initial Teasdale et al. (2000) trial results. Specifically, for those with severe childhood trauma, 41% of those who had MBCT relapsed, compared with 65% for those who had been allocated to TAU. The results for CPE were almost exactly in the middle: 54%. For those who had not experienced childhood trauma, the rates of relapse did not differ from each other: 51%, 45%, and 43% for MBCT, CPE, and TAU, respectively (Figure 18.2b).

When we computed the hazard ratio of relapse ("hazard ratio" is an index of risk over the time interval of follow-up, equivalent to a risk ratio if the follow-up period is identical for all), we found that for patients receiving MBCT the hazard ratio was 0.43 compared to those receiving TAU alone and 0.61 compared to those receiving CPE. *This*

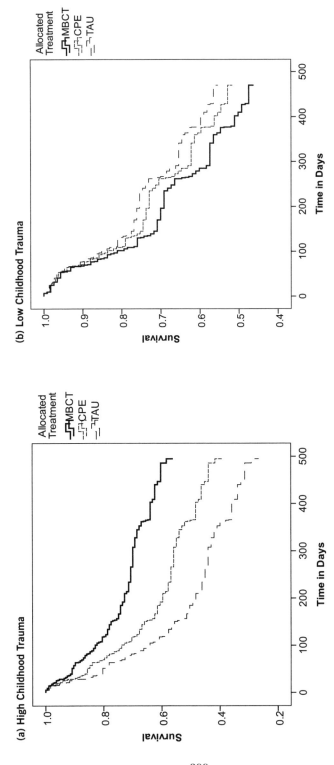

FIGURE 18.2. Proportions of patients who survived without relapse during follow-up in those with (a) high (n = 126) and (b) low (n, 129) Childhood Trauma Questionnaire scores. TAU, treatment as usual; CPE, cognitive psychoeducation + TAU; MBCT, mindfulness-based cognitive therapy + TAU.

means that MBCT reduces the chance of relapse by 57% compared to Treatment As Usual, and by 39% (1 minus 0.61) compared to cognitive psychoeducation. This means that overall MBCT is more effective in preventing relapse to major depression than both CPE and treatment as usual when severity of childhood trauma is taken into account. These results have been reported in detail in the *Journal of Consulting and Clinical Psychology* (Williams et al., 2014; see *www.oxfordmindfulness.org.science*).

Uncoupling Depression and Suicidal Thoughts and Urges

The "differential activation" model of suicidal reactivity on which our research program was based was outlined in Part I. The theory suggests that suicidal ideation originally arises as a feature of negative thinking during early episodes of depression (Williams et al., 2005). During these episodes, associations are formed between depressed mood, hopelessness and despair, and suicidal ideas. Now, in other periods of depressed mood (however the depression is caused) these patterns of thinking become active again. In this way, suicidal despair becomes folded in to the pattern of associations and feedback loops within the mind and body, and is reactivated and rehearsed with each subsequent episode of depression. We reviewed the evidence that suggested that after several episodes of suicidal depression, the return of low mood, even mild low mood, is sufficient to reinstate these habitual (suicidal) patterns and urges (Williams et al., 2005, 2006).

In our analyses we explored whether suicidal tendencies had reduced as the result of treatment. This analysis included even those people who became depressed again. Furthermore, we were interested to see whether either of the treatments had the effect of uncoupling the old habitual reactivation links between low mood and suicide. For this latter purpose we looked at relations specifically in those who showed mild to moderate symptoms at the end of the treatment. We used David Rudd's SCS (see p. 85), which defines suicidal despair in terms of Unlovability, Helplessness, and Poor Distress Tolerance.

The results were clear: MBCT had a larger effect on reducing suicidal despair than the other two groups, even when we took into account any changes in levels of depression. More importantly, when we investigated the relation between depressive symptoms and suicidal cognitions in patients with levels of symptoms that would normally be quite likely to trigger suicidal cognitions, we found that, while there were significant correlations between the strength of depressive symptoms and suicidal cognitions in the CPE and TAU groups, this was not the case in the MBCT group. This is an important result. It suggests that *following MBCT, suicidal cognitions are less likely to increase as depressive symptoms reoccur.*

The Role of Regular Practice

A main aim of the trial was to test the assumption that meditation practice is a crucially important component for reducing risk for relapse. We had offered a treatment (CPE) that was like MBCT in all respects except that it had no meditation practice included. We had found it was not so effective as full MBCT.

If actual meditation practice is important, then it implies that, even within the full MBCT groups, the more participants engage in the practice, the more they should reduce their risk for relapse. Participants had been asked to practice 6 days out of 7 each week and to keep diaries. We found that participants who reported that they engaged in formal home practice on at least 3 days a week during the treatment phase were almost half as likely to relapse as those who reported fewer than 3 days of formal practice. Overall 39% of those who practiced on 3 or more days per week relapsed over 12 months follow-up in comparison to 58% of those who practiced on less than 3 days per week. Again, our findings clearly suggested that practice does matter. But there is a problem in interpreting any such correlation between amount of practice and impact on depression. Even if a study finds that more practice is associated with better outcomes, it might be caused by a third factor: the enthusiasm of a participant for mindfulness. In treatment research, it is often found that participants who are better motivated because they believe in the theory behind it—so have high expectations of the intervention—have better outcomes. This is true whether or not any homework is involved. High expectation—believing that a treatment is credible—can be healing in itself. So could it be that those who come to MBCT with high expectations have better outcomes anyway. If so, they may well do more home practice but it may be the high expectation that is the hidden factor affecting *both* practice and the outcome. Recall that we had assessed participants' expectations (see "Treatment Credibility," above). This means that we could check to see if participants' expectations of MBCT predicted how well people fared and whether those with high estimate of treatment credibility did more home practice. The results were very clear. Unexpectedly, MBCT participants with higher expectations of MBCT did *not* do more home practice during the 8 weeks, and there was no association at all between this early expectation and eventual outcome. This shows that, *no matter how enthusiastic (or not) a participant was about MBCT at the beginning of the course, it was the actual amount of regular formal home practice that mattered.*

Reflections

We had conducted the largest trial of MBCT versus TAU to date, and the first to compare MBCT with an active psychological control treatment. A strength of the study was that we had very high rates of attendance at treatment sessions, with more than 90% of participants completing four or more sessions, which previous trials had judged an adequate minimum "dose" of treatment. The trial also had low rates of dropout, with only 7% of participants failing to give follow-up data. As we noted in Chapter 5, this was very different from the 30% dropout in our pilot work, and we could celebrate the effort that the whole team put into helping our participants right through the trial.

The findings that the more vulnerable patients were those with a history of childhood trauma and that it was this group that benefited from MBCT is consistent with previous results from MBCT trials. Our results are in line with the emerging picture that *MBCT is particularly helpful for those people who are at the greatest risk of relapse or recurrence.* Our research deliberately focused on people with a history of suicidal ideation or behavior, and it is known that childhood trauma is a particularly salient risk factor in this population (Williams et al., 2012). So we cannot claim from our study that it will always be childhood trauma that is the critical aspect of vulnerability. Exactly which patients are the most vulnerable differs across the different studies and will no doubt differ from clinic to clinic in different parts of the world. Some will be vulnerable because they had an early age of onset, others because they have experienced a larger number of episodes. Still others will be vulnerable because their mood is unstable even when they are not "clinically" depressed, and others because they suffered from trauma in childhood. The evidence to date, from several studies, suggests that researchers and clinicians first have to discern which participants in their own clinic are more vulnerable—for it is these people who are likely to benefit most from MBCT.

Implications

This trial brought to an end our 10-year program of research to understand suicidal depression and to see whether mindfulness training offered a way of preventing it. Looking to the future, what implications do our results have theoretically and practically for other applications of mindfulness?

First, the fact that the effects of CPE were intermediate between MBCT and TAU suggests that some of the effect of MBCT may be explained by the psychological education and group support provided by both MBCT and CPE interventions. However, our results suggest that simply coming to a class (experiencing a group atmosphere, a good teacher, and psychoeducation) are not enough. Mindfulness needs to be cultivated through the daily practice of formal and informal mindfulness practice. *The benefit of being aware is not just a good idea, it needs to be experienced and cultivated.* The fact that the amount of meditation practice participants engaged in during the course was significantly related to whether they relapsed or not during the 1-year follow-up further emphasizes this point.

Note, second, that we were investigating the prevention of recurrent suicidal depression, and so these results may not generalize to other groups of vulnerable people. Nevertheless, the pattern of results does suggest that whether mindfulness-based interventions are being offered for chronic pain, for cancer patients, for those with chronic anxiety, or for chronic health conditions, the question "Is it suitable for those of my patients who have had a traumatic childhood?" can be answered more confidently. It is not just our own results that point in this direction: *all* the trials that find that MBCT prevents depressive relapse point to the fact that it particularly helps those who have the longest history of psychological problems—very often associated with adverse childhood and adolescent experience.

Note, third, that it is not just the number of prior episodes, but the vulnerability that comes from being highly reactive to small changes in mood, that is critical. This implies that if these processes can be identified early—even before the first episode of depression—mindfulness could perhaps help people to steer themselves onto a completely different trajectory. Consistent with this idea, two recent exploratory trials of mindfulness for teenagers delivered as a universal intervention in schools found reduction in depression and increase in well-being (Kuyken et al., 2013), and a halving of new onsets of depression (Raes, Griffith, Van der Gucht, & Williams, 2014).

Finally, we need to take account of an important omission. One consequence of our focus on recurrent depression is that we did not assess positive emotions and "savoring." In a seminal study, Geschwind *did* include assessment of this using Experience Sampling in which people are sent reminders at random times during the day to answer a few questions about what they are doing, whether it is pleasant, and whether they are enjoying it (Geschwind, Peeters, Drukker, van Os, & Wichers, 2012). In a study of patients with residual symptoms, she found that MBCT increased such positive experiences, and that the degree to which it had this beneficial effect predicted clinical outcome. Because we did not assess this in our study, we now feel that we may have missed a very important aspect of mindfulness. For we know that mindfulness not only allows people to "let go" of negative aspects of the past and take a more decentered stance toward negative aspects of experience, but also helps people to reengage with life: to reclaim a sense of being intimately connected to small moment-to-moment beauties and pleasures that had long since seemed to disappear from their lives. People feel more awake, more alive. *We* assessed whether they felt less depressed, but future studies should follow Geschwind's example and also assess people's well-being, their "experience of being alive." This may also give us an answer to a paradox: MBCT seems, in these clinical studies, clearly to favor the most vulnerable, and not to be so effective for the less vulnerable. What is going on here?

MBCT for Those Who Are Not as Vulnerable

Here's the paradox: in people with a history of clinical depression, when MBCT is offered through a mental health clinic, it is most effective for participants whose difficulties are most severe. Yet thousands of MBCT and MBSR classes are offered all over the world for people who have never experienced an episode of depression, a trauma, or any serious psychological problem, and they report enormous benefit (see, e.g., Krusche, Cyhlarova, King, & Williams, 2012; Krusche, Cyhlarova, & Williams, 2013). How can this be?

Here is one possible answer. In most of the trials for recurrent depression there are many people with high vulnerability in the class. In this case it is inevitable that much of the attention is drawn to discussion of the high reactivity that arises from instability of mood and intrusion of traumatic memories. Those participants whose depression is less severe, or whose depression is a normal reaction to a major "life event," do not have these severe ruminative–reactivity problems, so focusing on them is less relevant for them. Furthermore, and this is where Geschwind's results may really help to clarify things, when there are more people in a class who are highly vulnerable, less of the class time is spent on the engagement and rediscovery of the small beauties and pleasures of life. By contrast, in a class where the majority are less vulnerable, there is much more opportunity to focus on the aspects of mindfulness that reveals the extraordinary power of simply "waking up." In classes with less vulnerable people, the patterns of mind that are focused on are those that *interfere with* engagement with the full flowering of moment-to-moment living, not patterns that are so toxic that they threaten to overwhelm the person at any moment. This can only be a tentative hypothesis at the moment, but will be an important and highly practical issue for future research to clarify.

Concluding Remarks

We have come to the end of our story. To summarize our results, the Oxford–Bangor collaboration showed that MBCT, offered when people feel well, may have particular beneficial effects in preventing future episodes of major depression, and may be especially relevant for those at highest risk of relapse. Particularly significant was our finding that MBCT "uncouples" mood from suicidal ideas and urges that it would have usually evoked.

The entire Wellcome Project started in 2003 with the idea that reactivation of suicidal ideas and behavior by small shifts in mood is at the center of why people remain vulnerable to suicidal depression. For our patients to begin to see that it does not have to be that way—for them to have the actual *experience* that sadness can come and go without producing a cascade of toxic thoughts and feelings—this in itself is extraordinarily liberating.

We are enormously grateful to the participants in all our research studies in Oxford, and those who took part in the Oxford–Bangor collaborative study, for it is through their willingness to participate that we are able to go forward with confidence. Through their efforts, we, as mindfulness teachers, need not be afraid of inviting those with the most difficult events in their past to take part in mindfulness training; and those seeking help can practice mindfulness with a deep sense of assurance, even if they have the most difficult life experience, that they are no longer need remain on the outside of life, looking in, but that here, now is a life worth living, truly and freely available to them.

Further Reading and Resources

How to Teach?

While the current book was written with practicing mindfulness teachers in mind, it is possible that you do not yet feel competent to teach it, and are wondering how to go about getting the necessary experience.

In this section, we reiterate much from Segal et al. (2013).

Starting Your Own Practice of Mindfulness

A central message in Segal et al. (2013) was that in order to do this work, therapists should practice mindfulness themselves. The best way is to be taught face-to-face by an experienced meditation teacher. However, if you first want to try it out for yourself, the best way is to work through the 8 weeks of *The Mindful Way Workbook* (Teasdale et al., 2014), using the downloads of guided meditation instructions that are included with it. The guidance will not only help you establish a regular practice but also provide a direct sampling of the exercises used by participants in the program (for other materials, see *http://oxfordmindfulness.org/learn/resources* or *www.bangor.ac.uk/mindfulness/ books.php.en*). Then, later, for more detailed description of the science behind the program, and the way it is taught session by session in class, see Segal et al. (2013).

Finding a Teacher

Segal and colleagues point out that there are many different forms of medita-
tion, so to prepare yourself as a potential instructor of MBCT, you need to
choose a tradition and teacher that are compatible in spirit and form with the
MBCT program: the Westernized insight meditation tradition. Information
about these centers can be obtained from the following: in North America,
Insight Meditation Society in Barre, Massachusetts (*www.dharma.org*) or Spirit
Rock in Woodacre, California (*www.spiritrock.org*); in Europe, Gaia House in
Devon, England (*www.gaiahouse.co.uk*); and in Australia *www.dharma.au*. In
addition, you may find a teacher from those centers that train mindfulness
teachers (see below).

Training Guidelines for MBCT Instructors

If, after you have sampled mindfulness for yourself, you are interested in
teaching mindfulness in a mental health setting, you will need to find training in the approach. Any training that does not insist on an established personal practice of mindfulness as a prerequisite of teaching, and that lasts
less than a year, is not going to give you the necessary basis for beginning to
offer this approach to your participants or clients. *This is true even if you are
an experienced therapist, and/or have sat many retreats.* Our experience of training many thousands of healthcare professionals all over the world to become
MBCT/MBSR teachers is that while therapy or retreat experience may help,
it may also hinder you in many subtle ways, so neither of these can ensure
that you are able to teach mindfulness.

In the United Kingdom, postgraduate training leading to a master's
degree in MBCT is available at Oxford University and the University of Exeter,
while Bangor University offers a masters in mindfulness, with both MBSR
and MBCT as a major focus. All of these U.K. based programs are taught on
a part-time basis over 2–4 years to professionals and provide coverage of the
experiential and didactic elements of MBCT, along with its evidence base.
There are other training centers being founded that are offering part or all of
these components; see the U.K. network at *http://mindfulnessteachersuk.org.uk*.

As Segal et al. (2013) indicate, a more likely scenario for instructors outside the United Kingdom or Europe, especially those living in North America,
is that you find yourself attending an MBCT clinical workshop, a silent mindfulness retreat for therapists, seeking supervision from a practicing MBCT
instructor, and then attending a peer supervision group. To help you chart
how far along you are in the process, Segal et al. give a roadmap—a list of what
they consider to be the normal minimal requirements for teaching MBCT for

mood disorders (see "Training Guidelines for Teaching MBCT," based on the U.K. Consensus Guidelines for Mindfulness Teachers, on pp. 310–311; to keep yourself up to date with these, see *http://mindfulnessteachersuk.org.uk/ pdf/MBI-TACJune2012.pdf*).

For further information, go to *www.bangor.ac.uk/mindfulness* and *www. oxfordmindfulness.org*, where there are many links to training opportunities and other resources to support your practice. In North America, you may find it helpful to look first at the centers at the University of Massachusetts (*www.umassmed.edu/cfm/training*) and the University of California, San Diego (*http://health.ucsd.edu/specialties/mindfulness*). In Australia, go to *www.mtia. org.au*; in Hong Kong, go to *www.mindfulness.hk/en/home*. Finally, there is a European network of training centers that you can access at *http://eamba.net*.

Further Reading to support Teachers and Participants

Segal, Z. V, Williams, J. M. G., & Teasdale, J. D. (2013). *Mindfulness-based cognitive therapy for depression* (2nd ed.). New York: Guilford Press.

This is the MBCT manual, essential reading for those who wish to teach MBCT to people suffering from mental health problems, but also proving helpful information to many other teachers of mindfulness who wish to understand the psychological theory that underlies and motivates the modern applications of mindfulness to emotional problems.

Teasdale, J., Williams, M., & Segal, Z. (2014). *The mindful way workbook.* New York: Guilford Press.

This book was written specifically to accompany participants as they work their way through the 8-week MBCT program. Along with describing the content in each session, participants are provided with a rationale for the different exercises and helpful hints for their growing practice. It is designed to function as single source for the handouts, home practice sheets, calendars, poems, CDs, and other content that is covered during the 8 weeks, and is *an essential resource to accompany this book.*

Williams, M., Teasdale, J., Segal, Z., & Kabat-Zinn, J. (2007). *The mindful way through depression: Freeing yourself from chronic unhappiness.* New York: Guilford Press.

This book is proving very helpful for people who are interested in reading about how the practice of mindfulness can be broadened to deal with milder, but more ubiquitous mental states, such as worry and unhappiness. It features guided meditations narrated by Jon Kabat-Zinn and provides the reader with more extensive background to these practices than would be typically provided in an MBCT class.

Williams, M., & Penman, D. (2011). *Mindfulness: Finding peace in a frantic world.* **London: Piaktus; New York: Rodale.**

This offers another option for those who wish to taste shorter meditation practices to see if this is something that they wish to explore further through the full MBCT program. It includes meditations narrated by Mark Williams (see *www.oxfordmindfulness.org*).

Crane, R. (2009). *Mindfulness-based cognitive therapy: Distinctive features.* **London: Routledge.**

A very useful general overview and introduction to the distinctive aspects of MBCT for teachers and prospective participants.

Silverton, S. (2012). *The mindfulness breakthrough: The revolutionary approach to dealing with stress, anxiety, and depression.* **London: Watkins.**

An illustrated introduction to mindfulness designed to be easily accessible for the general public and offering chapters exploring mindfulness within a range of life situations and specific conditions, including depression.

Free Podcast

The New Psychology of Depression is a series of six free podcasts by Mark Williams available from *iTunes-U*. It gives the background to depression in general, and how mindfulness works in reducing risk. Go to *https://itunes.apple.com/gb/itunes-u/new-psychology-depression/id474787597?mt=10*.

Training Guidelines for Teaching MBCT (from Segal, Williams, and Teasdale, 2013, p. 422)

These are normal minimal requirements for teaching MBCT for mood disorders.

1. An ongoing commitment to a personal mindfulness practice through daily formal and informal practice.
2. A professional qualification in clinical practice and mental health training that includes the use of structured, evidence based therapeutic approaches to affective disorders (e.g., cognitive behavioral therapy, interpersonal psychotherapy, ACT, behavioral activation).

3. Knowledge and experience of the populations that the mindfulness-based approach will be delivered to, including experience of teaching, therapeutic, or other care provision with groups and individuals.

4. Completion of an in-depth, rigorous mindfulness-based teacher training program or supervised pathway with a minimum duration of 12 months. (A "supervised pathway" might include attending three 8-week courses, the first as participant, the second as trainee, the third as coteacher, as well as attending workshops on theoretical and practical aspects of teaching the core practices and curriculum.)

5. Ongoing adherence to the framework for ethical conduct as outlined within his or her profession.

6. Engagement in an ongoing peer supervision process with an experienced *mindfulness-based teacher(s)* which includes:

7. Receiving periodic feedback on teaching from an experienced mindfulness-based teacher through video recordings, supervisor sitting in on teaching sessions or coteaching, and building in feedback sessions.

For the purposes of continuing professional development we recommend:

1. Participation in residential teacher-led mindfulness meditation retreats.

2. Ongoing peer supervision with mindfulness-based *colleagues*, built and maintained as a means to share experiences and learn collaboratively.

3. Engagement in *further training* to develop skills and understanding in delivering mindfulness-based approaches, including keeping up to date with the current evidence base for mindfulness-based approaches.

References

Appleby, L., Dennehy, J. A., Thomas, C. S., Faragher, E. G., & Lewis, G. (1999). Aftercare and clinical characteristics of people with mental illness who commit suicide: A case–control study. *Lancet, 353*, 1397–4000.

Anderson, R. J., Goddard, L., & Powell, J. H. (2010). Reduced specificity of autobiographical memory as a moderator of the relationship between daily hassles and depression. *Cognition and Emotion, 24*, 702–709.

Baer, R. (2003). Mindfulness training as a clinical intervention: A conceptual and empirical review. *Clinical Psychology: Science and Practice, 10*(2), 125–143.

Barnhofer, T., Duggan, D., Crane, C., Hepburn, S., Fennell, M. J. V., & Williams, J. M. G. (2007). Effects of meditation on frontal alpha-asymmetry in previously suicidal individuals. *NeuroReport, 18*, 709–712.

Bateman, A., & Fonagy, P. (2008). 8–year follow-up of patients treated for borderline personality disorder: Mentalization-based treatment versus treatment as usual. *American Journal of Psychiatry, 165*, 631–639.

Beautrais, A. L., Joyce, P. R., Mulder, R. T., Fergusson, D. M., Deavoil, B. J., & Nightingale, S. K. (1996). Prevalence and comorbidity of mental disorders in persons in serious suicide attempts: A case–control study. *American Journal of Psychiatry, 153*, 1009–1014.

Beck, A. T., Brown, G., Berchick, R. J., Stewart, B. L., & Steer, R. A. (1990). Relationship between hopelessness and ultimate suicide: A replication with psychiatric outpatients. *American Journal of Psychiatry, 147*, 190–195.

Beck, A. T., Rush, A. J., Shaw, B. F., & Emery, G. (1979). *Cognitive therapy for depression*. New York: Guilford Press.

Beck, A. T., Steer, R. A., & Brown, G. K. (1996). *Manual for the BDI-II*. San Antonio, TX: Psychological Corporation.

Beck, A. T., Weissman, A., Lester, D., & Trexler, L. (1974). The measurement of pessimism: The Hopelessness Scale. *Journal of Consulting and Clinical Psychology, 42*, 861–865.

Beiling, P., Hawley, L., Corcoran, K., Bloch, R., Levitan, R., Young, T., et al. (2012). Mediators of treatment efficacy in mindfulness-based cognitive therapy, antidepressant pharmacotherapy or placebo for prevention of depressive relapse. *Journal of Consulting and Clinical Psychology, 80,* 365–372.

Bernstein, D. P., & Fink, L. (1998). *Childhood Trauma Questionnaire: A retrospective self-report manual.* San Antonio, TX: Psychological Corporation.

Bernstein, D. P., Fink, L., Handelsman, L., Foote, J., Lovejoy, M., Wenzel, K., et al. (2003). Development and validation of a brief screening version of the Childhood Trauma Questionnaire. *Child Abuse and Neglect, 27*(2), 169–190.

Bodhi, B. (2011). What does mindfulness really mean?: A canonical perspective. *Contemporary Buddhism, 12*(1), 19–39.

Brewin, C. R., Gregory, J. D., Lipton, M., & Burgess, N. (2010). Intrusive images in psychological disorders: Characteristics, neural mechanisms, and treatment implications. *Psychological Review, 117*(1), 210–232.

Bockting, C. L. H., Schene, A. H., Spinhoven, P., Koeter, H. W. J., Wouters, L. F., Huyser, J., et al. (2005). Preventing relapse/recurrence in recurrent depression with cognitive therapy: A randomized controlled trial. *Journal of Consulting and Clinical Psychology, 73,* 647–657.

Bondolfi, G., Jermann, F., Van der Linden, M. V., Gex-Fabry, M., Bizzini, L., Weber Rouget, B., et al. (2010). Depression relapse prophylaxis with mindfulness-based cognitive therapy: Replication and extension in the Swiss health care system. *Journal of Affective Disorders, 122,* 224–231.

Brodsky, B. S., Oquendo, M., Ellis, S. P., Haas, G. L., Malone, K. M., & Mann, J. J. (2001). The relationship of childhood abuse to impulsivity and suicidal behavior in adults with major depression. *American Journal of Psychiatry, 158*(11), 1871–1877.

Brown, G. K., Have, T. T., Henriques, G. R., Xie, S. X., Hollander, J. E., & Beck, A. T. (2005). Cognitive therapy for the prevention of suicide attempts: A randomized controlled trial. *Journal of the American Medical Association, 294*(5), 563–570.

Burch, V. (2008). *Living well with pain and illness: Using mindfulness to free yourself from suffering.* London: Piatkus.

Carver, C. S., Lawrence, J. W., & Scheier, M. F. (1999). Self-discrepancy and affect: Incorporating the role of feared selves. *Personality and Social Psychology Bulletin, 25,* 783–792.

Collins, P. Y., Patel, V., Joestl, S. S., March, D., Insel, T. R., & Daar, A. S. (2011). Grand challenges in global mental health. *Nature, 475*(7354), 27–30.

Coryell, W., & Young, E. A. (2005). Clinical predictors of suicide in primary major depressive disorder. *Journal of Clinical Psychiatry, 66*(4), 412–417.

Cougle, J. R., Keough, M. E., Riccardi, C. J., & Sachs-Ericsson, N. (2009). Anxiety disorders and suicidality in the National Comorbidity Survey-Replication. *Journal of Psychiatric Research, 43*(9), 825–829.

Crane, C., Barnhofer, T., Duggan, D. S., Eames, C., Hepburn, S., Shah, D., & Williams, J. M. G. (2014). Comfort from suicidal cognition in recurrently depressed patients. *Journal of Affective Disorders, 155*(1), 241–246.

Crane, C., Barnhofer, T., Duggan, D. S., Hepburn, S., Fennell, M. J. V., & Williams, J. M. G. (2008). Mindfulness-based cognitive therapy and self-discrepancy in recovered depressed patients with a history of depression and suicidality. *Cognitive Therapy & Research, 32*, 775–787

Crane, C., Barnhofer, T., Visser, C., Nightingale, H., & Williams, J. M. G. (2007). The effects of analytical and experiential rumination on autobiographical memory specificity in individuals with a history of major depression. *Behaviour Research and Therapy, 45*, 3077–3087.

Crane, C., Shah, D., Barnhofer, T., & Holmes, E. A. (2012). Suicidal imagery in a previously depressed community sample. *Psychology and Psychotherapy, 19*(1), 57–69.

Crane, C., & Williams, J. M. G. (2010). Factors associated with attrition from mindfulness-based cognitive therapy in patients with a history of suicidal depression. *Mindfulness, 1*, 10–20.

Crane, R. S. (2009). *Mindfulness-based cognitive therapy: Distinctive features.* London: Routledge.

Crane, R. S., Eames, C., Kuyken, W., Hastings, R. P. L., Williams, J. M. G., Bartley, T., et al. (2013). Development and validation of the Mindfulness-Based Interventions—Teaching Assessment Criteria (MBI:TAC). *Assessment, 20*(6), 681–688.

Crane, R. S., & Kuyken, W. (2012), The implementation of mindfulness-based cognitive therapy: Learning from the UK Health Service experience. *Mindfulness, 4*(3), 246–254.

Crane, R. S., Soulsby, J. G., Kuyken, W., Williams, J. M. G., & Eames, C. (2012). *The Bangor, Exeter and Oxford Mindfulness-Based Interventions Teaching Assessment Criteria (MBI-TAC) for assessing the competence and adherence of mindfulness-based class-based teaching.* Bangor University. Retrieved January 30, 2014, from *www.bangor.ac.uk/mindfulness/documents/MBI-TACJune2012.pdf.*

Danese, A., & McEwen, B. S. (2012). Adverse childhood experiences, allostasis, allostatic load, and age-related disease. *Physiology and Behavior, 106*(1), 29–39.

Dalgleish, T., Williams, J. M. G., Golden, A.-M. J., Perkins, N., Feldman Barrett, L., Barnard, P. J., et al. (2007). Reduced specificity of autobiographical memory and depression: The role of executive control. *Journal of Experimental Psychology: General, 136*, 23–42.

Debeer, E., Raes, F., Williams, J. M. G., & Hermans, D. (2011). Context dependent activation of reduced autobiographical memory specificity as an avoidant coping style. *Emotion, 11*, 1500–1506.

Dreyfus, H. L., & Dreyfus, S. E. (1986). *Mind over machine: The power of human intuition and experience in the age of computers.* New York: Free Press.

Duggan, D. (2008). *Psychological mechanisms underlying suicidal behavior.* Unpublished D. Phil thesis, University of Oxford.

Ehlers, A., & Clark, D. M. (2000). A cognitive model of posttraumatic stress disorder. *Behaviour Research and Therapy, 38*(4), 319–345.

Evans, A., Crane, R. S., Cooper, L., Mardula, J., Wilks, J., Surawy, C., et al. (2014, March 23). A framework for supervision for mindfulness-based teachers: A space for embodied mutual inquiry. *Mindfulness* [online publication].

Felder, J. N., Dimidjian, S., & Segal, Z. (2012). Collaboration in mindfulness-based cognitive therapy. *Journal of Clinical Psychology: In Session, 68*(2), 179–186.

First, M. B., Spitzer, R. L., Gibbon, M., & Williams, J. B. W. (2002). *Structured Clinical Interview for DSM-IV-TR Axis I Disorders, Research Version, Patient Edition (SCID-I/P)*. New York: Biometrics Research, New York State Psychiatric Institute.

Geschwind, N., Peeters, F., Drukker, M., van Os, J., & Wichers, M. (2011) Mindfulness training increases momentary positive emotions and rewards experience in adults vulnerable to depression: A randomized controlled trial. *Journal of Consulting and Clinical Psychology, 79*, 618–628.

Gibbs, B. R., & Rude, S. S. (2004). Overgeneral autobiographical memory as depression vulnerability. *Cognitive Therapy and Research, 28*, 511–526.

Gilbert, P. (1989). *Human nature and suffering*. Hove, UK: Erlbaum.

Godfrin, K. A., & van Heeringen, C. (2010). The effects of mindfulness-based cognitive therapy on recurrence of depressive episodes, mental health and quality of life: A randomized controlled study. *Behaviour Research and Therapy, 48*, 738–746.

Gordon, K. H., Selby, E. A., Anestis, M. D., Bender, T. W., Witte, T. K., Braithwaite, S., et al. (2010). The reinforcing properties of repeated deliberate self-harm. *Archives of Suicide Research, 14*(4), 329–341.

Gould, M., Marrocco, F. A., Kleinman, M., Thomas, J. G., Mostkoff, K., Cote, J., et al. (2005). Evaluating iatrogenic risk of youth suicide screening programs: A randomized controlled trial. *Journal of the American Medical Association, 293*(13), 1635–1643.

Hargus, E., Hawton, K., & Rodham, K. (2009). Distinguishing between subgroups of adolescents who self-harm. *Suicide and Life-Threatening Behavior, 39*(5), 518–537.

Hawton, K., Casañas, I., Comabella, C., Haw, C., & Saunders, K. (2013). Risk factors for suicide in individuals with depression: A systematic review. *Journal of Affective Disorders, 147*, 17–28.

Hayes, S. C., Strosahl, K., Wilson, K. G., Bissett, R. T., Pistorello, J., Toarmino, D., et al. (2004). Measuring experiential avoidance: A preliminary test of a working model. *Psychological Record, 54*(4), 553–578.

Heeren, A., Van Broeck, N., & Philippot, P. (2009). The effects of mindfulness on executive processes and autobiographical memory specificity. *Behaviour Research and Therapy, 47*, 403–409.

Heim, C. M., Mayberg, H. S., Mletzko, T., Nemeroff, C. B., & Pruessner, J. C. (2013). Decreased cortical representation of genital somatosensory field after childhood sexual abuse. *American Journal of Psychiatry, 170*(6), 626–623.

Hepburn, S. R., Crane, C., Barnhofer, T., Duggan, D. S., Fennell, M. J. V., & Williams, J. M. G. (2009). Mindfulness-based cognitive therapy may reduce thought suppression in previously suicidal participants: Findings from a preliminary study. *British Journal of Clinical Psychology, 48*(2), 209–215.

Hollon, S. D., DeRubeis, R. J., Shelton, R. C., Amsterdam, J. D., Salomon, R. M., O'Reardon, J. P., et al. (2005). Prevention of relapse following cognitive therapy vs. medications in moderate to severe depression. *Archives of General Psychiatry, 62*, 417–422.

Hollon, S. D., & Kendall, P. C. (1980). Cognitive self-statements in depression: Development of an Automatic Thoughts Questionnaire. *Cognitive Therapy and Research, 4*(4), 383–395.

Holmes, E. A., Crane, C., Fennell, M. J. V., & Williams, J. M. G. (2007). Imagery about suicide in depression—"flash-forwards"? *Behaviour Therapy and Experimental Psychiatry, 38 (4),* 423–434.

Holmes, E. A., & Mathews, A. (2005). Mental imagery and emotion: A special relationship? *Emotion, 5*(4), 489–497.

Ingram, R. E., Miranda, J., & Segal, Z. V. (1998). *Cognitive vulnerability to depression.* New York: Guilford Press.

Inskipp, F., & Proctor, B. (1995). *The art, craft, and tasks of counselling supervision: Part 1. Making the most of supervision.* Twickenham, UK: Cascade.

Joiner, T. E., Rudd, M. D., & Rajab, M. H. (1997). The Modified Scale for Suicidal Ideation: factors of suicidality and their relation to clinical and diagnostic variables. *Journal of Abnormal Psychology, 106,* 260–265.

Kabat-Zinn, J. (2013). *Full catastrophe living* (rev. ed.). New York: Bantam Books.

Kahneman, D. (2012). *Thinking fast and slow.* London: Penguin Books.

Katz, C., Yaseen, Z. S., Mojtabai, R., Cohen, L. J., & Galynker, I. (2011). Panic as an independent risk factor for suicide attempts in depressive illness: Findings from the National Epidemiological Survey on Alcohol and Related Conditions (NESARC). *Journal of Clinical Psychiatry, 72*(12), 1625–1635.

Kendler, K. S., Gardner, C. O., & Prescott, C. A. (1999). Clinical characteristics of major depression that predict risk of depression in relatives. *Archives of General Psychiatry, 56*(4), 322–327.

Kendler, K. S., Thornton, L. M., & Gardner, C. O. (2001). Genetic risk, number of previous episodes, and stressful life events in predicting onset of major depression. *American Journal of Psychiatry, 158*(4), 582–586.

Kidger, J., Heron, J., Lewis, G., Evans, J., & Gunnell, D. (2012). Adolescent self-harm and suicidal thoughts in the ALSPAC cohort: A self-report survey in England. *BMC Psychiatry, 12,* 69.

Krusche, A., Cyhlarova, E., King, S., & Williams, J. M. G. (2012). Mindfulness online: A preliminary evaluation of the feasibility of a web-based mindfulness course and the impact on stress. *BMJ Open, 2*(3), e000803.

Krusche, A., Cyhlarova, E., & Williams, J. M. G. (2013). Mindfulness online: An evaluation of the feasibility of a web-based mindfulness course for stress, anxiety and depression. *BMJ Open, 3*(11), e003498.

Kuyken, W., Weare, K., Ukoumunne, O. C., Vicary, R., Motton, N., Burnett, R., et al. (2003). Effectiveness of the mindfulness in schools programme: Non-randomised controlled feasibility study. *British Journal of Psychiatry, 203*(2), 126–131.

Libby, L. K., Shaeffer, E. M., Eibach, R. P., & Slemmer, J. A. (2007). Picture yourself at the polls: Visual perspectives in mental imagery affects self-perception and behavior. *Psychological Science, 18*(3), 199–203.

Linehan, M. M. (1993). *Cognitive-behavioral treatment of borderline personality disorder.* New York: Guilford Press.

Linehan, M. M., Goodstein, J. L., Nielsen, S. L., & Chiles, J. A. (1983). Reasons for staying alive when you are thinking of killing yourself: The Reasons for Living Inventory. *Journal of Consulting and Clinical Psychology, 51*(2), 276–286.

MacLeod, A. K., Pankhania, B., Lee, M., & Mitchell, D. (1997). Parasuicide, depression, and the anticipation of positive and negative future experiences. *Psychological Medicine, 27*(4), 973–977.

Ma, S. H., & Teasdale, J. D. (2004). Mindfulness-based cognitive therapy for depression: Replication and exploration of differential relapse prevention effects. *Journal of Consulting and Clinical Psychology, 72*(1), 31–40.

MacLeod, A. K., Rose, G., & Williams, J. M. G. (1993). Components of hopelessness about the future in parasuicide. *Cognitive Therapy & Research, 17*, 441–455.

McCown, D., Reibel, D., & Micozzi, M. S. (2010). *Teaching mindfulness: A practical guide for clinicians and educators*. New York: Springer.

Miranda, J., & Persons, J. B. (1988). Dysfunctional attitudes are mood state dependent. *Journal of Abnormal Psychology, 97*, 76–79.

Miller, A. (2007). *The drama of the gifted child: The search for the true self*. New York: Basic Books.

Mondimore, F. M., Zandi, P. P., MacKinnon, D. F., McInnis, M. G., Miller, E. B., Schweizer, B., et al. (2007). A comparison of the familiality of chronic depression in recurrent early-onset depression pedigrees using different definitions of chronicity. *Journal of Affective Disorders, 100*(1–3), 171–177.

National Institute for Health and Care Excellence. (2009a). *Borderline personality disorder* (Clinical Guideline 78). London: Author.

National Institute for Health and Care Excellence. (2009b). *Depression: The treatment and management of depression in adults* (Clinical Guideline 90). London: Author.

National Institute for Health and Care Excellence. (2011). *Self-harm: Longer-term management* (Clinical Guideline CG133). London: Author.

Nolen-Hoeksema, S., Wisco, B. E., & Lyubomirsky, S. (2008). Rethinking rumination. *Perspectives on Psychological Science, 3*, 400–424.

O'Connor, R. C. (2003). Suicidal behaviour as a cry of pain: Test of a psychological model. *Archives of Suicide Research, 7*, 297–308.

O'Connor, R. C. (2011). Towards an integrated motivational-volitional model of suicidal behaviour. In R. C. O'Connor, S. Platt, & J. Gordon (Eds.), *International handbook of suicide prevention: Research, policy and practice* (pp. 181–198). Chichester, UK: Wiley–Blackwell.

O'Connor, R. C., O'Carroll, R. E., Ryan, C., & Smyth, R. (2012). Self-regulation of unattainable goals in suicide attempters: A two year prospective study. *Journal of Affective Disorders, 142*, 248–255.

O'Connor, R. C., O'Connor, D. B., O'Connor, S. M., Smallwood, J. M., & Miles, J. (2004). Hopelessness, stress and perfectionism: The moderating effects of future thinking. *Cognition and Emotion, 18*, 1099–1120.

Oquendo, M. A., Currier, D., & Mann, J. J. (2006). Prospective studies of suicidal behavior in major depressive and bipolar disorder: What is the evidence for predictive risk factors? *Acta Psychiatrica Scandinavica, 114*, 151–158.

Orbach, I., Mikulincer, M., Gilboa-Schechtman, E., & Sirota, P. (2003). Mental pain and its relationship to suicidality and life meaning. *Suicide and Life-Threatening Behavior, 33*(3), 231–241.

Orbach, I., Mikulincer, M., Sirota, P., & Gilboa-Schechtman, E. (2003). Mental pain: A multi-dimensional operationalization and definition. *Suicide and Life-Threatening Behavior, 33*(3), 219–230.

Palmer, P. J. (1997). The heart of a teacher identity and integrity in teaching. *Change: The Magazine of Higher Learning, 29*(6), 14–21.

Parker, G., Roussos, J., Hadzi-Pavlovic, D., Mitchell, P., Wilhelm, K., & Austin, M.-P. (1997). The development of a refined measure of dysfunctional parenting and assessment of its relevance in patients with affective disorders. *Psychological Medicine, 27*(5), 1193–1203.

Parker-Palmer. (1983). *To know as we are known: A spirituality of education.* San Francisco: Harper & Row.

Piet, J., & Hougaard, E. (2011). The effect of mindfulness-based cognitive therapy for prevention of relapse in recurrent major depressive disorder: A systematic review and meta-analysis. *Clinical Psychology Review, 31*, 1032–1040.

Platt, J. J., Spivak, G., & Bloom, W. (Eds.). (1978). *Manual for the Means–End Problem Solving (MEPS) Procedure: A measure of interpersonal problem-solving skill.* Philadelphia: Hahnemann Medical College Hospital.

Pollock, L. R., & Williams, J. M. G. (1998). Problem solving and suicidal behavior. *Suicide and Life-Threatening Behavior, 28*(4), 375–387.

Pollock, L. R., & Williams, J. M. G. (2001). Effective problems solving in suicide attempters depends on specific autobiographical recall. *Suicide and Life-Threatening Behavior, 31*(4), 386–396.

Price, J. S., & Sloman, L. (1987). Depression as yielding behavior: An animal model based on Schjelderup-Ebbe's pecking order. *Ethology and Sociobiology, 8*(Suppl. 10), 855–985.

Raes, F., Griffith, J. W., Van der Gucht, K., & Williams, J. M. G. (2014). School-based prevention and reduction of depression in adolescents: A cluster-randomized controlled trial of a mindfulness group program. *Mindfulness, 5*, 477–486.

Rawal, A., Williams, J. M. G., & Park, R. (2011). Effects of analytical and experiential self-focus on stress-induced cognitive reactivity in eating disorder psychopathology. *Behaviour Research and Therapy, 49*(10), 635–645.

Rawal, A., & Rice, F. (2012). Examining overgeneral autobiographical memory as a risk factor for adolescent depression. *Journal of the American Academy of Child and Adolescent Psychiatry, 51*, 518–527.

Rihmer, Z. (2001). Can better recognition and treatment of depression reduce suicide rates?: A brief review. *European Psychiatry, 16*(7), 406–407.

Rudd, M. D., Joiner, T., & Rajab, M. H. (2001). *Treating suicidal behavior: An effective, time-limited approach.* New York: Guilford Press.

Rycroft-Malone, J., Anderson, R., Crane, R. S., Gibson, A., Gadinger, F., Owen Griffiths, H., et al. (2014). Accessibility and implementation in UK services of an effective depression relapse prevention program—Mindfulness-based cognitive therapy (MBCT): ASPIRE study protocol. *Implementation Science, 9*, 62.

Santorelli, S. (1999). *Heal thy self.* New York: Bell Tower.

Santorelli, S., Goddard, T., Kabat-Zinn, J., Kesper-Grossman, U., & Reibel, D. (2011). *Standards for the formation of MBSR teacher trainers: Experience, qualifications, competency and ongoing development.* Paper presented at the Investigating and Integrating Mindfulness in Medicine, Health Care, and Society 9th Annual International Scientific Conference, Worcester, MA.

Salzberg, S. (1995). *Lovingkindness: The revolutionary art of happiness.* Boston: Shambhala.

Schmidt, N. B., Woolaway-Bickel, K., & Bates, M. (2001). Evaluating panic-specific factors in the relationship between suicide and panic disorder. *Behaviour Research and Therapy, 39,* 635–649.

Segal, Z. V., Bieling, P., Young, T., MacQueen, G., Cooke, R., Martin, L., et al. (2010). Antidepressant monotherapy vs. sequential pharmacotherapy and mindfulness-based cognitive therapy, or placebo, for relapse prophylaxis in recurrent depression. *Archives of General Psychiatry, 67*(12), 1256–1264.

Segal, Z. V., Gemar, M., & Williams, S. (1999). Differential cognitive response to a mood challenge following successful cognitive therapy or pharmacotherapy for unipolar disorder. *Journal of Abnormal Psychology, 108*(1), 3–10.

Segal, Z. V., Kennedy, S., Gemar, M., Hood, K., Pedersen, R., & Buis, T. (2006). Cognitive reactivity to sad mood provocation and the prediction of depressive relapse. *Archives of General Psychiatry, 63,* 749–755.

Segal, Z. V., Williams, J. M. G., & Teasdale, J. D. (2002). *Mindfulness-based cognitive therapy for depression (1st ed.): A new approach to preventing relapse.* New York: Guilford Press.

Segal, Z. V., Williams, J. M. G., & Teasdale, J. D. (2013). Mindfulness-based cognitive therapy for depression (2nd ed.). New York: Guilford Press.

Segal, Z. V., Williams, J. M. G., Teasdale, J. D., & Gemar, M. C. (1996). A cognitive science perspective on kindling and episode sensitization in recurrent affective disorder. *Psychological Medicine, 26,* 371–380.

Sharpless, B. A., & Barber, J. P. (2009). A conceptual and empirical review of the meaning, measurement, development, and teaching of intervention competence in clinical psychology. *Clinical Psychology Review, 29,* 47–56.

Shea, S. C. (1999). *The practical art of suicide assessment: A guide for mental health professionals and substance abuse counselors.* New York: Wiley.

Shneidman, E. S. (1985). *Definition of suicide.* New York: Wiley.

Sinclair, J., Cranc, C. K., Hawton, K., & Williams, J. M. G. (2007). The role of autobiographical memory specificity in deliberate self-harm: Correlates and consequences. *Journal of Affective Disorders, 102,* 11–18.

Stange, J. P., Hamlat, E. J., Hamilton, J. L., Abramson, L. Y., & Alloy, B. L. (2013). Overgeneral autobiographical memory, emotional maltreatment, and depressive symptoms in adolescence: Evidence of a cognitive vulnerability stress interaction. *Journal of Adolescence, 36,* 201–208.

Stengel, E. (1964). *Suicide and attempted suicide* (rev. ed.). Harmondsworth, UK: Penguin Books.

Sumner, J. A., Griffith, J. W., Mineka, S., Newcomb Rekart, K., Zinbarg, R. E., & Craske, M. G. (2011). Overgeneral autobiographical memory and chronic interpersonal stress as predictors of the course of depression in adolescents. *Cognition and Emotion, 25,* 183–192.

Taylor, S., Zvolensky, M. J., Cox, B. J., Deacon, B., Heimberg, R. G., Ledley, D. R., et al. (2007). Robust dimensions of anxiety sensitivity: Development and initial validation of the Anxiety Sensitivity Index–3. *Psychological Assessment, 19*(2), 176–188.

Teasdale, J. D. (1988). Cognitive vulnerability to persistent depression. *Cognition and Emotion, 2,* 247–274.

Teasdale, J. D. (1999). Emotional processing: Three modes of mind and the prevention of relapse in depression. *Behaviour Research and Therapy, 37*(Suppl. 1), S53–S77.

Teasdale, J. D., Moore, R. G., Hayhurst, H., Pope, M., Williams, S., & Segal, Z. V. (2002). Metacognitive awareness and prevention of relapse in depression: Empirical evidence. *Journal of Consulting and Clinical Psychology, 70,* 275–287.

Teasdale, J. D., Segal, Z. V., & Williams, J. M. G. (1995). How does cognitive therapy prevent relapse and why should attentional control (mindfulness) training help? *Behaviour Research and Therapy, 33,* 225–239.

Teasdale, J. D., Segal, Z. V., Williams, J. M. G., Ridgeway, V. A., Soulsby, J. M., & Lau, M. A. (2000). Prevention of relapse/recurrence in major depression by mindfulness-based cognitive therapy. *Journal of Consulting and Clinical Psychology, 68*(4), 615–623.

Teasdale, J. D., Williams, J. M. G., & Segal, Z. V. (2014). *The mindful way workbook: An 8-week program to free yourself from depression and emotional distress.* New York: Guilford Press.

Treynor, W., Gonzalez, R., & Nolen-Hoeksema, S. (2003). Rumination reconsidered: A psychometric analysis. *Cognitive Therapy and Research, 27*(3), 247–259.

UK Network for Mindfulness-Based Teacher Training Organisations. (2011). *Good practice guidance for teaching mindfulness-based courses.* Retrieved January 30, 2014, from *http://mindfulnessteachersuk.org.uk.*

Van der Does, A. J. W. (2002). Cognitive reactivity to sad mood: Structure and validity of a new measure. *Behaviour Research and Therapy, 40*(1), 105–120.

Van der Does, A. J. W., & Williams, J. M. G. (2003). *Leiden Index of Depression Sensitivity–Revised.* Leiden University. Retrieved from *www.dousa.nl/publications_depression.htm?LEIDS.*

Van Orden, K. A., Witte, T. K., Cukrowicz, K. C., Braithwaite, S. R., Selby, E. A., & Joiner, T. E. (2010). The interpersonal theory of suicide. *Psychological Review, 117,* 575–600.

Watkins, E. (2008). Constructive and unconstructive repetitive thought. *Psychological Bulletin, 134,* 163–206.

Watkins, E., & Moulds, M. (2005). Distinct modes of ruminative self-focus: Impact of abstract versus concrete rumination on problem solving in depression. *Emotion, 5*(3), 319–328.

Wegner, D. M. (1994). Ironic processes of mental control. *Psychological Review, 101,* 34–52.

Wegner, D. M., & Zanakos, S. (1994). Chronic thought suppression. *Journal of Personality, 62*(4), 616–640.

Wells, A. (2009) *Metacognitive therapy for anxiety and depression.* New York: Guilford Press.

Williams, J. M. G. (1997). *Cry of pain* (1st ed.): *Understanding suicide and self-harm.* London: Penguin Books.

Williams, J. M. G. (2008). Mindfulness, depression and modes of mind. *Cognitive Therapy and Research, 32,* 721–733.

Williams, J. M. G. (2014). *Cry of pain* (updated and expanded ed.): *Understanding suicide and the suicidal mind.* London: Piatkus.

Williams, J. M. G., Alatiq, Y., Crane, C., Barnhofer, T., Fennell, M. J. V., Duggan, D. S., et al. (2008). Mindfulness-based cognitive therapy (MBCT) in bipolar disorder: Preliminary evaluation of immediate effects on between-episode functioning. *Journal of Affective Disorders, 107,* 275–279.

Williams, J. M. G., Barnhofer, T., Crane, C., & Beck, A. T. (2005). Problem solving deteriorates following mood challenge in formerly depressed patients with a history of suicidal ideation. *Journal of Abnormal Psychology, 114,* 421–431.

Williams, J. M. G., Barnhofer, T., Crane, C., Duggan, D. S., Shah, D., Brennan, K., et al. (2012). Pre-adult onset and patterns of suicidality in patients with a history of recurrent depression. *Journal of Affective Disorders, 138*(1–2), 173–179.

Williams, J. M. G., Barnhofer T., Crane, C., Herrman, D., Raes, F., Watkins, E., et al. (2007). Autobiographical memory specificity and emotional disorder. *Psychological Bulletin, 133*(1), 122–148.

Williams, J. M. G., Crane, C., Barnhofer, T., Brennan, K., Duggan, D. S., Fennell, M. J. V., et al. (2014). Mindfulness-based cognitive therapy for preventing relapse in recurrent depression: A randomized dismantling trial. *Journal of Consulting and Clinical Psychology, 82,* 275–286.

Williams, J. M. G., Crane, C., Barnhofer, T., Van der Does, A. J. W., & Segal, Z. V. (2006). Recurrence of suicidal ideation across depressive episodes. *Journal of Affective Disorders, 91*(2–3), 189–194.

Williams, J. M. G., Duggan, D. S., Crane, C., & Hepburn, S. (2011). Modes of mind and suicidal processes: The potential role of mindfulness in changing minds. In R. C. O'Connor, S. Plath, & J. Gordon (Eds.), *International handbook of suicide prevention: Research, policy, and practice* (pp. 401–418). Chichester, UK: Wiley.

Williams, J. M. G., Teasdale, J. D., Segal, Z. V., & Soulsby, J. (2000). Mindfulness-based cognitive therapy reduces overgeneral autobiographical memory in formerly depressed patients. *Journal of Abnormal Psychology, 109*(1), 150–155.

Williams, J. M. G., Van der Does, A. J. W., Barnhofer, T., Crane, C., & Segal, Z. V. (2008). Cognitive reactivity, suicidal ideation and future fluency: Preliminary investigation of a differential activation theory of hopelessness/suicidality. *Cognitive Therapy and Research, 32*(1), 83–104.

Williams, J. M. G., Watts, F. N., MacLeod, C., & Mathews, A. (1997). *Cognitive psychology and emotional disorders.* Chichester, UK: Wiley.

World Health Organization. (2008). *The global burden of disease: 2004 update.* Geneva, Switzerland: Author.

Zisook, S., Rush, A. J., Lesser, I., Wisniewski, S. R., Trivedi, M., Husain, M. M., et al. (2007). Preadult onset vs. adult onset of major depressive disorder: A replication study. *Acta Psychiatrica Scandinavica, 115*(3), 196–205.

Index

List of Audio Files

Track	Title	Run Time
1	Welcome and Introduction	00:57
2	Raisin Exercise	09:53
3	Body Scan	39:08
4	10-Minute Sitting Meditation—Mindfulness of the Breath	09:54
5	Mindful Movement—Formal Practice	38:30
6	Stretch and Breath Meditation	33:39
7	Mindful Walking	13:42
8	3-Minute Breathing Space—Regular Version	05:02
9	3-Minute Breathing Space—Responsive Version	05:19
10	20-Minute Sitting Meditation	20:38
11	Sitting Meditation	37:47
12	Working with Difficulty Meditation	25:47
13	Bells at 5 Minutes, 10 Minutes, 15 Minutes, 20 Minutes, and 30 Minutes	30:32

Terms of Use